3/10

DISEASES IN HISTORY
HIV/AIDS

Diseases
in History

HIV/AIDS

Kevin Cunningham

MORGAN
REYNOLDS

PUBLISHING

Greensboro, North Carolina

Diseases in History

PLAGUE

FLU

MALARIA

HIV/AIDS

DISEASES IN HISTORY: HIV/AIDS

Copyright © 2009 By Kevin Cunningham

Library of Congress Cataloging-in-Publication Data

Cunningham, Kevin, 1966-
  Diseases in history. HIV/AIDS / by Kevin Cunningham.
    p. cm.
  Includes bibliographical references and index.
  ISBN-13: 978-1-59935-104-9
  ISBN-10: 1-59935-104-8
  1. AIDS (Disease)--History. I. Title. II. Title: HIV/AIDS.
  RC606.6.C86 2009
  614.5'99392--dc22

                                    2008051616

Printed in the United States of America
First Edition

Contents

Introduction

One of the worst disease-related disasters in human history is happening today.

Since 1981, human immunodeficiency virus, or HIV, has infected an estimated 65 million people worldwide. Approximately 33 million people carried HIV at the end of 2007.

Twenty-five million have died.

Unlike most infectious diseases, HIV works at a very slow pace. It takes years—sometimes seven or eight, even ten or twelve—for symptoms to show up. All during that time, however, it pulverizes the human immune system. Eventually, the body cannot fight off even minor infections. Unusual conditions show up: a form of pneumonia caused by a common bacterium. Severe, even disfiguring, genital sores. A rare form of cancer. Ravaging tuberculosis.

At that point, the infected person has the advanced condition caused by HIV—acquired immunodeficiency syndrome, or AIDS.

Technically, no one dies of AIDS. Victims actually die of the infections that take advantage of the immune system's inability to fight.

After emerging from its isolated point of origin in the African rain forest, HIV spread slowly for decades, and in such shadowy ways we can only guess at most of its history.

But no infectious disease rains down on humanity out of nowhere.

All have been (and are) assisted by human behavior. The link between behavior and illness is in no way unique to HIV and AIDS. Humans have always created conditions agreeable to pathogens, going back to prehistory, when people domesticated animals and started sharing their microbes, and forward to the filthy cities of the Middle Ages that encouraged plague-bearing rats, and forward again to the exhausted laborers of the 1800s who gasped for air with lungs consumed by tuberculosis.

HIV thrived on promiscuity and poverty, took advantage of our modern forms of transportation, secretly rode in blood supplies shipped around a country or around the world.

Two types of HIV circulate in humans. The less common form, HIV-2, originated in a virus carried by a species of African monkey. Though a serious disease, HIV-2 progresses to AIDS more slowly than the virus's other form. HIV-2 is mostly seen in West Africa, in former Portuguese colonies in other parts of Africa, and in Mumbai, India.

HIV-1 had its origins in a virus carried by chimpanzees. When this book refers to HIV, it refers to HIV-1. Due to its habit of mutating into new forms, HIV-1 has split off into several genetically distinct categories of viruses called clades. The "B" clade causes most HIV infections in the United States. The "E" clade dominates in Southeast Asia. To keep things clear, this book uses "HIV" as an umbrella term for all of them.

The history of HIV is short, but as varied as the countries stricken, indeed as varied as the individuals infected. In many ways it parallels the epidemics of the past. In other ways, it does not. In all ways, it's been an extraordinary, if horrible, historical event. As one report put it:

> Throughout history, few crises have presented such a threat to human health and to social and economic progress as does the HIV/AIDS epidemic. This is even more troubling given the realization that much of the suffering and destitution caused by the disease could have been prevented.

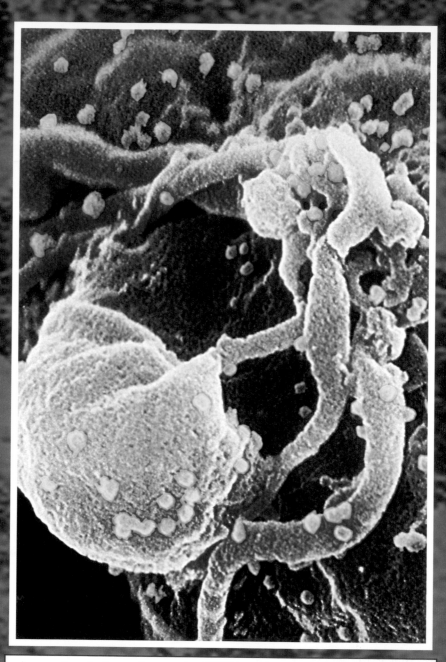

A scanning electron micrograph of HIV (seen here as rounded green bumps) on a lymphocyte. *(Courtesy of Centers for Disease Control and Prevention)*

one

The Virus

For the most part, the major infectious diseases we're familiar with have caused humanity problems for centuries. Human immunodeficiency virus (HIV), however, apparently crossed over to human beings from animals in the recent past. Genetic tests by scientists at Los Alamos National Laboratory point to a date around 1931.

"There's no reason to believe this was just lingering around in people," said Beatrice Hahn, a University of Alabama-Birmingham scientist studying the origin of AIDS.

HIV has a relative in the animal world called simian immunodeficiency virus, or SIV. Different types of SIV occur in different species of primates. A chimpanzee SIV labeled SIVcpz was the ancestor of the more common of the two human immunodeficiency viruses, HIV-1—the virus that leads to AIDS in the vast majority of cases around the world.

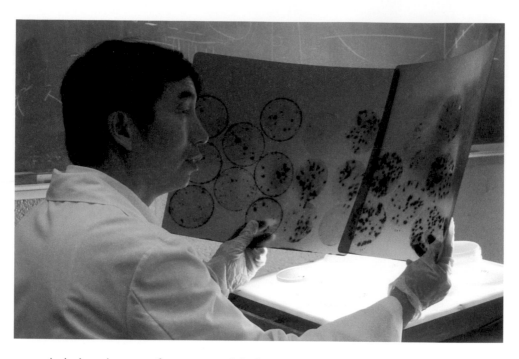

A simian virus was the ancestor of the human immunodeficiency virus. In this 1985 photo, a scientist compares a simian virus to HIV-1. *(Courtesy of National Cancer Institute)*

SIVcpz may have circulated in chimps for a long time. Advanced laboratory tests have shown that chimpanzees in Cameroon's remote rain forests continue to be infected with a form of SIVcpz that is genetically similar to HIV.

Around 1931, some event took place—we're still not sure what—that caused SIVcpz to mutate into a virus capable of infecting, and killing, human beings.

How humans first caught HIV may never be known. One popular theory suggests that hunters came into contact with the blood of an infected chimp. A bite or scratch from an animal could have introduced the virus. It's just as possible, however, that it was transmitted in uncooked meat, from a tame chimp to its owner, or in some other way.

The animal-to-human transfer of disease isn't unusual. A majority of the infectious diseases we deal with originated in animals. Influenza, for example, probably crossed over from ducks.

The mutated virus we now call HIV possibly infected African villagers in whatever area (or areas) it originated. At times it may have hit a dead end and vanished without infecting large numbers of people, only to leap from chimps to humans at another time to start a new chain of infections.

Eventually, HIV began to circulate among human beings. It passed between people in small numbers at first. Then it accelerated in the population until it caused an epidemic, a dramatic term that really just means an above-average number of cases of a disease in an area or country.

An unusual virus caused this epidemic. HIV is a lentivirus (slow virus), a genus within the retrovirus family. Retroviruses, like HIV itself, are relatively new to us. A great deal of the research on them began only in the 1970s. Then, scientists thought retroviruses (and by extension lentiviruses) only caused disease in nonhuman mammals like cats and sheep.

As the name implies, the slow virus HIV infects a person for years before signs of disease appear. This trait is one of HIV's most devastating weapons. A person has no idea he or she is infected and unknowingly spreads the virus to others for years.

A particle of HIV resembles a sphere studded with plunger-shaped proteins. Inside the particle, a cylindrical core holds two strands of ribonucleic acid, or RNA, coded with the virus's nine genes. Copies of other proteins important to the virus also float around the core.

Besides working on a slow schedule, human immunodeficiency virus has one other unusual trait. It constantly changes its genetic structure.

In HIV, the structural change takes place because the virus codes its genes on RNA. A virus coded in deoxyribonucleic acid, or DNA, has a mechanism for making sure it copies itself accurately. RNA operates without that editor, so it makes mistakes in the copying process. The imperfect copies are known as mutations.

Over time, mutation has caused HIV to split into a group of related but diverse viruses. As of the year 2000, there were twenty-four known families of HIV. Together, those families contained more than a thousand forms of HIV. Each of these

This illustration shows how HIV invades a T-cell and replicates itself by depositing and mutating viral RNA. *(Courtesy of National Cancer Institute)*

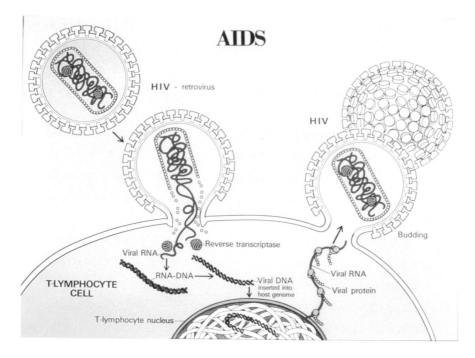

forms, or strains, qualifies as HIV. But their distinct genetic codes set them apart from the others.

HIV is extremely fragile. For that reason, the virus cannot pass through the air, nor by casual contact. Unlike influenza, for instance, it can't survive on a drinking glass or tabletop. It simply isn't able to live in the open air.

The virus's fragility limits the ways HIV can transmit itself from one person to the next.

An infected person can give it to a sex partner through unprotected vaginal, anal, or oral sex. HIV, despite its fragility, thrives in the tissues of the sex organs, the rectum, and to a lesser extent in the mouth. Breaks in the lining in these regions and sores from other infections increase the chance of passing on the virus. In new cases worldwide, sexual contact was the most common form of transmission.

HIV also spreads through blood. Infection via this method hits hardest at intravenous drug users who share needles and syringes. IV drug users fuel the virus's spread in many countries.

Related transmission routes include reusing needles for medical procedures (a problem in African countries), or unsafe blood donation practices (the cause of a major epidemic in China). In the days before blood companies tested for the virus, thousands of people contracted HIV through transfusions during surgery or related to the treatment of hemophilia, a genetic disorder.

Finally, mothers can pass HIV to newborn children. Drug treatments have all but eliminated this problem in the U.S. and other rich countries. But HIV-stricken mothers in the developing world often don't have access to the medicines. Infants can also get the virus through breast milk.

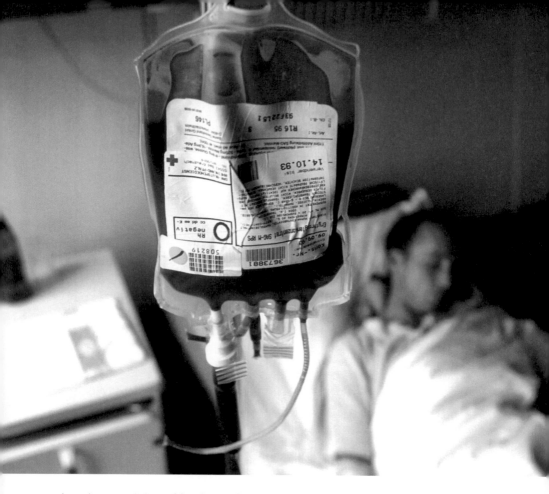

A patient receiving a blood transfusion in a hospital. HIV can be transmitted by unprotected sex, contact with infected blood, or from a mother to her child. *(Courtesy of Vario Images GmbH & Co.KG/Alamy)*

Some people newly infected with HIV experience a short bout with a flulike illness. Symptoms can include a persistent headache, fever, rash, swollen glands, or fatigue. Symptoms typically (but not always) appear two to four weeks after exposure to the virus, though it can happen in a matter of days or in rare cases up to six months later.

Because the symptoms are commonplace and because they usually last a few weeks at most, many fail to connect the seemingly mild illness to HIV infection. A person then enters a long asymptomatic phase. The length of this period varies.

An infected person may show the symptoms associated with advanced disease in a matter of months to three years after being infected. Usually, however, it takes something closer to eight or ten years.

The lack of symptoms doesn't mean the virus remains dormant. Once in the body, HIV multiplies fast. It immediately goes to work on cells connected to the immune system.

Until the AIDS epidemic, the immune system got a lot less attention than it does today. It's truly one of the miracles of the human body. As we walk through life, we encounter untold numbers of potentially harmful viruses, bacteria, parasites, and fungi. The various kinds of cells that make up the immune system detect, learn about, and destroy these invaders before any can take up residence in the body.

In a healthy person, the immune system succeeds virtually every time, despite being under constant attack. When it fails, we get sick.

T-cells are a group of immune cells that "learn" and "remember" the threats encountered by our body. If we encounter the same threat again, certain specialized T-cells help identify it and call for "hunter-killers" programmed to wipe out the invader.

This ferocious response is the reason a human gets the measles only once. After we get over measles the first time, our immune system can identify and destroy the measles virus whenever we encounter it.

HIV tampers with the way the immune system responds. It targets an important type of immunity cell known as the CD4 positive (CD4+) T-cells. CD4+ T-cells are sometimes called the conductor or quarterback of the immune system. They direct the orchestra or draw up the play, meaning they summon the hunter-killers of the immune system and coordinate the attack against an invading microbe.

Without CD4+ T-cells, the immune system is left leaderless and cannot function.

HIV attacks by latching onto a cell that carries the specific CD4+ molecule on its surface. The virus particle and cell then merge together. Having broken in, the virus infiltrates the cell's command center, the nucleus. It then employs an unusual ability to replace the cell's genetic "blueprint" with its own set of plans. In doing so it literally becomes part of the cell.

From that point on, the cell works for the virus, reproducing thousands of copies of the viral invader. HIV, once established, manufactures billions of new virus particles in a person each day.

The human immune system still destroys a great many of the HIV particles. But, inevitably, some escape. The body's immune cells learn to recognize some of the forms of HIV by locking in on its genetic markers. But they can't keep track of all the mutated versions created by the virus's imperfect copying software.

Thus, no matter how much the immune system learns, new versions of the virus always remain functional. Two versions can even swap genes and create yet another new, hybrid strain.

In addition to attacking the CD4+ T-cells, HIV damages the immune system by playing havoc with certain molecules that control our immunity response. Specialized immunity-related organs like the lymph nodes come under focused attack and break down, further hurting the body's ability to respond to invading microbes. The virus can also travel to the brain, creating severe neurological problems.

HIV also seems to hide in other types of immunity cells and in a small number of the undamaged CD4+ T-cells, as well. Since this reservoir of virus uses a hijacked cell as a hiding place, medication doesn't recognize it as an invader. For that reason, HIV always surges back, even when drugs seem to clear it from the body.

The destruction of CD4+ and other cells slowly undermines the immune system. As an infection advances, a person may lose an extreme amount of weight, suffer from fatigue and fever, and experience a variety of conditions like rashes, yeast infections, or severe herpes.

In time, the number of CD4+ T-cells fall to a level that makes it impossible for the immune system to mount an effective defense. A healthy person shows a level of about eight hundred to 1,200 of the CD4+ T-cells in a cubic millimeter of blood. The number falls as HIV spreads. The decline can be steady or sudden.

When a victim's CD4+ count drops below two hundred, doctors consider the person to have the advanced form of HIV infection—acquired immunodeficiency syndrome, or AIDS.

Not everyone with a count below two hundred shows symptoms. A majority do, however. Symptoms take the form of opportunistic infections. Many of the microbes causing these conditions are harmless to a healthy person because the immune system destroys them long before they cause illness.

But an immune system devastated by HIV, particularly when it has advanced to AIDS, leaves a person extraordinarily vulnerable.

The Centers for Disease Control recognize twenty-six conditions common to AIDS cases. The list includes certain cancers caused by viruses, like Kaposi's sarcoma and cancer of the cervix, as well as lymphomas (cancers of the immune system). AIDS also invites in diarrhea and other gastrointestinal problems; aggressive forms of herpes; tuberculosis, certain kinds of pneumonia, and other respiratory illnesses; brain infections; eye infections; fatigue; appetite loss; extreme weight loss; mental deterioration; lack of coordination; seizures; and coma.

Once a patient shows a CD4+ count associated with AIDS, or an AIDS-related opportunistic infection and HIV infection, doctors thereafter consider the person to have AIDS, regardless of any improvement that may follow.

In the early years of the epidemic, a person diagnosed with AIDS almost always died in less than two years. In the

Kaposi's sarcoma, a type of cancer caused by a virus, on the skin of an AIDS patient *(Courtesy of Centers for Disease Control and Prevention)*

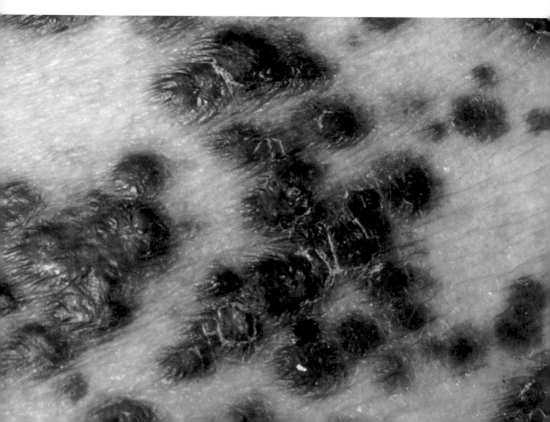

parts of the world without access to the treatment, that's still the case.

Today, thanks to breakthroughs with medicines, an HIV-positive person can live for years if he or she has access to treatment. Research also shows longer periods of survival in people who have progressed to AIDS.

Many things about HIV seemed new and alien when it first appeared. That it behaved in ways no one understood, for instance. That the first outbreaks appeared in places as far apart as the U.S. and Haiti and East Africa. That it only seemed to affect specific groups of people.

But the events that occurred once HIV crossed over to us had parallels in history. The first epidemics ravaged humanity as soon as people began to collect into cities thousands of years ago. Ever since, human behaviors of many kinds have played a role in the success (and once in a while the failure) of infectious diseases. Ever since, we have scrambled to react to every new adversary in a variety of ways—to understand it through science, to fight it with compassion and logic and faith, to assist its advance with arrogance and apathy and panic and bigotry.

So it was when the Black Death battered the medieval world. So it was when deadly influenza killed tens of millions in the early twentieth century. And so it was when a mysterious wasting illness turned up in far-flung locations at the end of the 1970s.

two
The Emerging Epidemic

T he earliest confirmed HIV infection dates from 1959. That year, a man in Kinshasa, a city in the Belgian Congo (today the Democratic Republic of Congo) gave a blood sample. Scientists testing it decades later detected HIV.

But there aren't a lot of facts to help researchers track HIV's progress after that.

Some researchers and historians believe it arrived in the United States around 1968, most likely several times with several carriers. How remains unclear.

According to one theory, Haiti linked the African virus with the U.S. strain. Haiti's HIV problem emerged around the same time the disease appeared in the U.S. Since AIDS symptoms took so long to show up, it was clear the virus had infected people in the Caribbean years earlier.

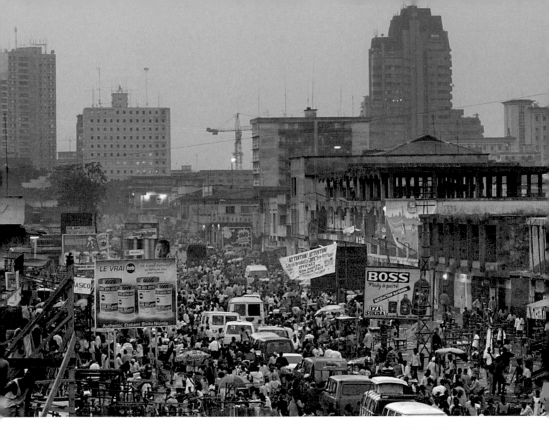

A view from a street in Kinshasa, the city in the Democratic Republic of Congo where the earliest confirmed HIV case was identified. *(Courtesy of AP Images)*

In the 1960s and 1970s, Haitians had gone to central Africa, including the former Belgian Congo, for jobs or to work as mercenaries. While there, the theory goes, these Haitians contracted HIV and brought it back home. It then took a decade for the first AIDS cases to show up. American tourists, in the meantime, caught the virus in Haiti and carried it to the U.S.

Another theory proposes that American travelers brought it back from Africa and, shortly thereafter, took it to Haiti.

Whatever happened, HIV took hold and spread in silence, its victims unaware they were infected, the people they gave it to just as unaware, and both, like everyone in the world, ignorant of the fact that anything like HIV even existed.

Then, around the mid-1970s, the number of people with the virus suddenly increased.

In 1978, sex workers in Port-au-Prince, Haiti's capital, began to fall ill with respiratory illness and rare cancers.

Around the same time, a handful of unusual cases turned up in doctors' offices in California and New York City. All the patients were young men. All were homosexual, or gay. All had infections that were either rare or so ordinary they shouldn't have caused medical problems.

Perhaps the most baffling condition was *Pneumocystis carinii* pneumonia. Almost everyone carries the *Pneumoystis* organism. It is one of the many ordinary bacteria in our bodies kept under control by the immune system.

Under normal circumstances, *Pneumocystis carinii* pneumonia, or PCP, only caused problems in people with immune systems damaged by cancer treatment or in elderly patients living in the close quarters of nursing homes.

In addition to PCP, patients dealt with one or many inexplicable ailments, including extreme weight loss, fatigue, and severe fungal infections.

The agents causing these conditions hadn't suddenly learned to elude the immune system of young Americans. Instead, the patients had immune systems so damaged that the men could no longer fight off supposedly harmless infections.

Michael Gottlieb, a doctor at the University of California at Los Angeles Medical Center, had treated some of these men. Along with his colleagues, Gottlieb reported five of the cases to the Centers for Disease Control (CDC) in Atlanta.

The CDC printed the report in the June 5, 1981, edition of its *Morbidity and Mortality Weekly Report*. Readers learned that two of the men—both previously healthy, one aged thirty-three, the other twenty-nine—had died. *Pneumocystis carinii* had shown up in their bodies.

The report, titled "Pneumocystis Pneumonia—Los Angeles," was the first appearance of HIV and AIDS in the medical literature. June 5 is now considered the anniversary of the start of the HIV/AIDS epidemic.

A month later, a second report appeared, this one dealing with cases of Kaposi's sarcoma, a rare kind of skin cancer caused by a virus. Like PCP, Kaposi's sarcoma had suddenly started turning up in young gay men.

As it turned out, the reports were related.

HIV emerged at a time of social upheaval in the United States. From the mid-1960s on, many Americans explored relationships and sexuality in a way unfathomable to previous generations, encouraged by easy access to birth control and a loosening of societal mores.

In purely biological terms, the so-called sexual revolution provided sexually transmitted diseases increased opportunities to infect new hosts. A person with multiple partners left himself open to increased risk of infection simply because more partners equaled more chances of catching something.

Syphilis, once in decline, roared back. Cytomegalovirus, a kind of herpes linked to cancer (and later to AIDS), infected more than 90 percent of the gay men living in some major cities.

Antibiotics took care of many of such infections. The rest were endured, as necessary, or treated, if possible.

Other upheavals roiled American society, as well. The gay liberation movement had begun in New York City in 1969 and spread quickly to gay communities in some major cities. Gay

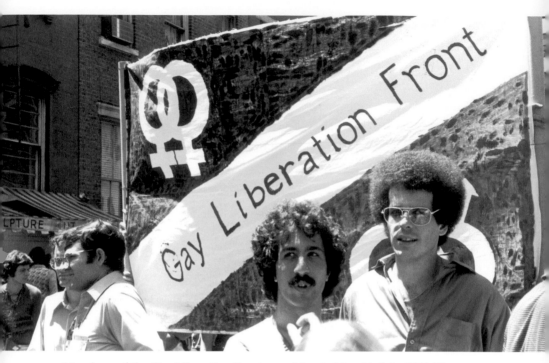

Members of the Gay Liberation Front marching in New York in 1970. The gay liberation movement began in New York City in 1969 and spread quickly to gay communities in other major cities. *(Courtesy of Getty Images)*

neighborhoods in San Francisco, New York, and a handful of other cities attracted thousands of men from all over the country, happy to live open ("out") lives where others approved of their sexual preference.

As San Francisco author Armistead Maupin recalled,

> The thing that annoys me most is the . . . attitude that gay people didn't discover the bonds of family until AIDS and death forced it upon them. Nothing could be further from the truth. There were, as early as the mid-seventies in San Francisco, gay lawyer groups, gay doctor groups, gay needlepoint groups, gay sports teams, and people forming viable, loving families.

With the mood of liberation in the air, sex for many gay men took on a political dimension. They used sex to build a sense of solidarity and as a declaration of their newfound freedom.

A small part of gay society embraced this idea to a fantastic degree. These men had hundreds of sex partners per year. Promiscuity, considered negative by large parts of society, became for them a badge of honor.

It also improved the chances of catching a sexually transmitted disease. HIV was the latest addition to the list.

In July 1981, the CDC created a task force to look into the Kaposi's sarcoma epidemic. By the end of the summer, researchers had identified 108 cases of severe immune system problems in gay men. They named the condition GRID, or gay-related immune deficiency. Its cause was unknown. The effects, however, were becoming clearer.

In a healthy human being, the immune system operates at peak efficiency from early adulthood through the mid-thirties. Yet GRID laid waste to the immune systems of this group in particular.

Once diagnosed with GRID, a patient often deteriorated at a rapid pace, their skin spotted with purple Kaposi's sarcoma lesions, gasping from pneumonia, nearly skeletal from rapid weight loss, bedridden with fatigue, stricken with seizures, hit all over the body by both common and bizarre infections. One physician described it as a "total body rot. It's merciless."

GRID patients had trouble getting treatment. The bewildering variety of related infections made it hard to diagnose. Very few physicians had seen GRID before. And information was scarce. A lot of the early reports on GRID appeared in the

CDC's *Morbidity and Mortality Weekly Report*, a publication read mostly by public health officials, not doctors.

Some people, even experts, doubted an infectious disease could foil modern medicine for long. In the twentieth century, science had invented vaccines, medicines, pesticides, and a host of other treatments that broke infectious diseases' hold, at least in wealthy nations. Polio, malaria, diphtheria, tetanus, scarlet fever, measles—all had been major health problems in the U.S. in the first half of the twentieth century. By 1980, all had come under control.

There was a widespread belief that, once science unlocked GRID's secrets, the disease would be defeated. "I think there was certainly the idea that this was a flash in the pan, that this was going to come and go and would die out," said one infectious disease specialist years later. "That little window of optimism didn't last long."

Research groups studied a number of viruses to determine what part each played, if any, in GRID. By June 1982, the available evidence pointed toward a sexually-transmitted virus carried in the blood: a virus, because antibiotics didn't work against it; and blood, because it partially explained the recent appearance of the disease in groups outside the gay community.

Of those groups, intravenous drug users appeared to be most affected.

Intravenous drug addiction had become a visible social problem in cities in the 1970s. Heroin, available in volumes never seen before, led the way. Where injecting the drug had once required a costly glass or steel syringe, plastic syringes and disposable needles now provided cheap alternatives.

Many intravenous drug users lived desperate lives, supporting their addictions with theft and prostitution, often living on the street or in shelters, too poor to spend three dollars on a clean needle, too fatalistic to think it worthwhile.

Those in urban areas often clustered in abandoned buildings, nicknamed shooting galleries, to inject. Addicts at a shooting gallery often shared syringes and needles to save money. Traces of blood from one person transmitted microbes in his bloodstream to anyone sharing.

Health professionals attempted to address the connection between the disease and the IV drug problem. Needle exchange programs seemed an obvious tool. Officials in a few European countries already handed out free needles so that users didn't risk exposure to the virus by sharing.

Needle exchanges ignited instant controversy in the U.S. African American clergy and community leaders, aware of what drugs had done to their neighborhoods, blasted the idea as encouraging drug use. "It's genocide, pure and simple," said one New York City councilman.

The public's worries about infected needles went beyond illegal drug use, however. Blood banks ran low because people feared they'd be exposed by giving blood. A handful of those able to afford it set up private blood banks for themselves and their families.

In addition to IV drug users, Haitian immigrants, people suffering from hemophilia, as well as small numbers of children, also showed signs of extreme breakdown in the immune system.

With the exception of children, and in addition to gay men, these categories became what public health officials referred to as risk groups—groups of people identified as at greater risk to catch a disease due to some combination of factors.

The label "risk group" wasn't intended to create prejudice. In fact, the concept was and is used for medical conditions across the board. Overweight people, for example, are a risk group when it comes to diabetes.

But the risk group label ended up being used as a weapon by those wishing to blame the disease on gays and by others eager to transfer the virus's origin, then thought to be in the U.S., to Haiti or elsewhere.

GRID had become an obsolete term when the disease appeared outside the gay community. In July 1982, a conference of government officials, researchers, gay activists, and others agreed to the more accurate description of acquired immunodeficiency syndrome. The CDC soon sent out guidelines to health care providers and laboratory workers on protecting one's self from AIDS patients and lab samples taken from them.

Research, meanwhile, showed that women had become a risk group. Physicians had reported that infected men, many of them IV drug users, were transmitting AIDS to women via sexual contact. Some doctors and scientists doubted the truth of such observations, or the accuracy of more recent reports that pregnant women had passed AIDS to their newborn children.

A lack of hard data drove the skepticism but so did fear. The implication that heterosexuals could catch the disease had terrifying implications for its spread.

By September 1983, AIDS cases in the U.S. and Puerto Rico numbered 2,259. The death rate approached 1,000. Sixteen months later, both numbers had tripled.

The gay community, while not solely affected, was hit hardest. Gay men watched in horror as friends, lovers, ex-lovers, partners, and community leaders died, often in the prime of life, often after devastating illness.

"I am angry and frustrated almost beyond the bound my skin and bones and body and brain can encompass," wrote playwright and activist Larry Kramer. "My sleep is tormented by nightmares and visions of lost friends, and my days are flooded by the tears of funerals and memorial services and seeing my sick friends. How many of us must die before all of us living fight back?"

A 1989 photo of playwright and AIDS activist Larry Kramer. *(Courtesy of Yale Collection of American Literature, Beinecke Rare Book and Manuscript Library)*

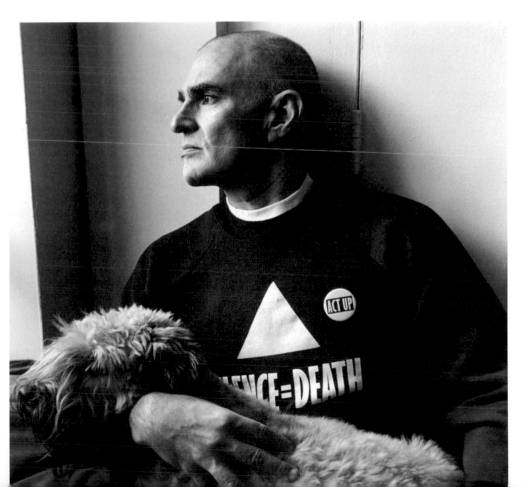

Statistics circulated that 86 percent of people diagnosed with late stage AIDS died. Very few major infectious diseases killed at that rate. A rise in suicide was reported among those diagnosed with the disease.

Physicians for the most part asked their gay patients to recognize the relationship between promiscuous sex and AIDS and change their habits, to save themselves but to also stop the disease from spreading. Many gays who had practiced promiscuity took the advice.

But a vocal minority condemned these men as traitors and sell-outs. To them, giving up any aspect of their sexuality—when they had been harassed, beaten, even arrested for it—was unacceptable. Arguments raged in the gay press about how to react to AIDS, about how to incorporate the disease into one's politics and sexual identity as well as one's lifestyle. These attitudes sometimes complicated a doctor's ability to treat a patient.

Scientists, meanwhile, searched for the cause. A team led by Robert Gallo of the National Institutes of Health had considered a retrovirus a likely culprit behind AIDS for some time. His theory startled peers. An AIDS-causing retrovirus would be a difficult opponent. Retroviruses were poorly understood. Their ability to turn the body's cellular machinery against itself would pose problems when the time came to develop medicines.

Gallo had done pioneering work on retroviruses in the 1970s and his opinions carried huge weight in the scientific community. By all accounts, he was brilliant. He had a shelf of awards to prove it.

He was also highly competitive—to a fault, some said. Critics had accused him of trumpeting research before the

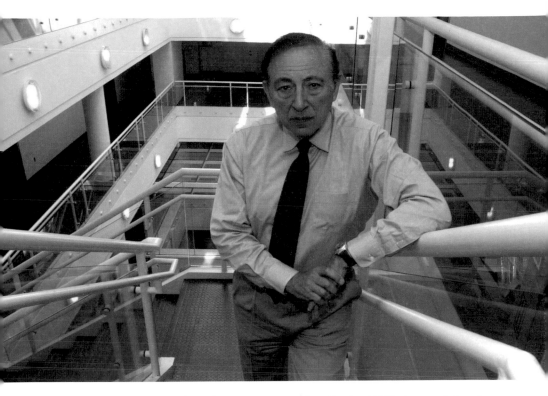

Dr. Robert Gallo was one of the first scientists to identify the AIDS virus and develop a test for the disease. *(Courtesy of AP Images/Gail Burton)*

results were in, of claiming work done by his staff as his own. Nonetheless, Gallo plunged into the search for AIDS's cause. He had already connected retroviruses to immunity problems and certain kinds of cancer. Seeing similarities, he boldly claimed one of two retroviruses he had discovered, or a still-unknown relative of same, was the agent behind AIDS.

Others worked on the puzzle as well. In 1983, Luc Montagnier, a scientist at Paris's Pasteur Institute, identified a new retrovirus that behaved differently than those studied by Gallo. Montagnier labeled his retrovirus lymphadenopa-thy associated virus, or LAV. Both he and Gallo published their results in the same issue of *Science,* a leading scientific journal. Neither claimed his virus caused AIDS, only that the research suggested a relationship between the agent in question and the disease.

The labs led by the two men collaborated on research even as they competed to find the cause of the disease. Montagnier became suspicious of foul play when Gallo claimed he had found a new retrovirus and that it definitely caused AIDS. It turned out Gallo's newest discovery was virtually the same as LAV. The French fumed as Gallo accepted credit as the discoverer of the AIDS virus.

LAV (soon to be renamed human immunodeficiency virus) did, in fact, cause AIDS. But that wasn't the end of the story. The U.S. government awarded Gallo and his colleagues a patent related to the virus, a financial gold mine that also implied Gallo had sole claim to the discovery. Montagnier sued.

A number of embarrassing revelations soon challenged Gallo's side of the story. Critics wondered if he had appropriated the French virus. The more forgiving assumed the French samples had contaminated Gallo's, a common danger in laboratory work.

In the end, and after much negotiation, the two scientists agreed to share the credit. Gallo later wrote a book telling his version of what happened. Montagnier went on to isolate the HIV-2 virus from West Africans.

In October 2008, Montagnier and fellow French researcher Francoise Barre-Sinoussi shared with German Harald zur Hausen the Nobel Prize in medicine, which cited the French scientists' discovery of HIV. Previously, Gallo had admitted that a lab error had contaminated his work with the French strain, and in 1994 the U.S. government granted France more royalties because Gallo had relied on the French virus.

But by the mid-1980s, the virus's discovery had already paid immediate benefits. Using the new knowledge, scientists developed tests to diagnose patients and to check for HIV in donated blood. Health authorities and blood products companies had known for a long time that HIV tainted the U.S. blood supply. That put hemophiliacs at particular risk of infection.

Victims of a genetic quirk that prevented their blood from clotting properly, hemophiliacs depended on periodic infusions of products derived from blood. Many used Factor VIII injections or infusions. Before Factor VIII and similar treatments, America's approximately 26,000 hemophiliacs lived, on average, until just past age eleven. After the treatments became available, the figure rose to age thirty-eight.

Manufacturers made Factor VIII from the blood of thousands of donors. In essence, a hemophiliac shared blood with every one of those people. If one donor in the pool had HIV, an entire batch of blood products might be tainted.

Blood companies and banks had guaranteed the safety of their products and the nation's blood supply. Scientists disagreed. Evidence had piled up that people in the hospital for surgery, as well as hemophiliacs, had contracted HIV through transfusions.

But companies complained that the research linking donated blood to HIV was inconclusive, that the costs of running tests on the entire blood supply were too high. Scientists and blood products businesses argued for months while the Food and Drug Administration, the government agency in charge of guaranteeing blood safety, chose to watch and wait.

As a result, tainted blood and blood products like Factor VIII infected thousands of Americans—the exact number is unknown—through treatment for hemophilia or transfusions during surgery and other medical procedures. Tennis star Arthur Ashe, a former Wimbledon and U.S. Open champion, got HIV during heart surgery. So did writer Isaac Asimov. Activist Elizabeth Glaser caught the virus after needing a blood transfusion while giving birth.

Tennis star Arthur Ashe contracted HIV after receiving infected blood during heart surgery. Before companies began testing donated blood for HIV, many people became infected after receiving tainted blood during medical procedures. *(Courtesy of Focus on Sport/Getty Images)*

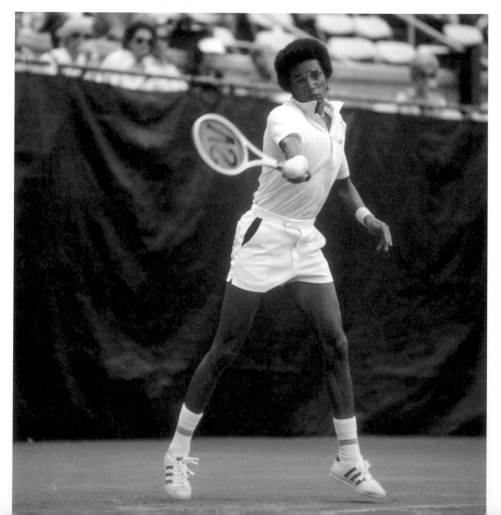

Technicians started using the new test on blood samples in late 1984. On March 2, 1985, it became available to the public. The test's manufacturer sent the first kits to the Irwin Memorial Blood Bank in San Francisco, the source of a considerable number of transfusion-related infections.

Blood tests provided a valuable weapon against infection, but the technology also opened up the possibility for darker uses. A Florida state health officer told colleagues at the CDC and Food and Drug Administration that he'd heard from school districts wanting to use the test to identify and fire gay teachers.

That kind of story may have reflected prejudice or genuine worry. But it illustrated the dilemma faced by public health officials. On the one hand, they knew tried and true ways to control an outbreak of infectious disease. On the other, they had to weigh whether those methods might violate the civil rights of patients.

Take quarantines. Removing infectious citizens from society had played a role in public health practice going back to the Black Death. Quarantines were forced on immigrants in Honolulu and San Francisco during plague outbreaks in the early 1900s. Authorities generally settled for a more voluntary system during the 1918–1919 influenza epidemic.

A few politicians and media figures floated the idea for AIDS patients. It never got beyond words. Gay activists and civil liberties groups argued vehemently against such proposals. Not surprisingly, gays were no more willing than any other American to be kept locked up, especially since AIDS, being an incurable illness, logically meant quarantine had to be permanent. The *New England Journal of Medicine* condemned the idea.

Mandatory testing for HIV in certain groups had much stronger government support. It also met similar resistance. Opponents claimed mandatory testing stepped on individual rights, especially since there was no legal guarantee the test results would remain private. As it was, an HIV-positive label could legally cost a person his job, home, and health insurance. Edwin Meese, the attorney general, had already ruled that a person could be fired if he or she was merely *thought* to have AIDS by co-workers.

Public health experts, unable or unwilling to use some of the old tools, turned to providing information as a major weapon against the disease. Brochures, pamphlets, comics, and posters spelled out the scientific facts on HIV and AIDS, advised drug users to use clean syringes and needles, and preached safe sex. Many were provided by HIV activists, social service groups, and medical organizations.

Condoms, a product no one dared advertise even a few years earlier, became one of the epidemic's iconic images. Pamphlets explained how to use them. Posters kept them in the public eye. Dance clubs and inner-city clinics and university health centers gave them away.

These kinds of programs, especially those funded with government money, inevitably generated controversy. Some thought the information went too far in discussing sex and drug use. Others thought it didn't go far enough. Arguments and accusations, and many lectures on morality, charged the atmosphere.

Then, an unlikely figure jumped in and attracted fire from both sides.

Before C. Everett Koop, the office of surgeon general was more ceremonial than anything else. Koop, famous for his

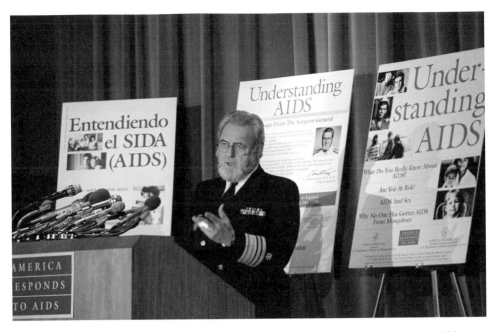

Surgeon General C. Everett Koop announcing that the federal government will be mailing a pamphlet on AIDS to every American household in 1988. *(Courtesy of AP Images)*

stern expression and his habit of dressing in the military-style uniform of the Public Health Service, changed that image. Regarded as reliably conservative at a time when conservatives were at odds with AIDS activists, he issued a report that shocked his political allies with its honesty.

Koop proposed that sex education be started in elementary school, stressed the need to teach teens about sexuality both at school and at home, and praised monogamy and abstinence while at the same time advocating condom use. He dismissed ideas to register HIV-positive people or quarantine them. While he supported testing, he said it had to take place alongside strong laws that promised privacy and prevented discrimination. Anything else, and people simply wouldn't get tested, a dangerous choice for themselves and others.

Koop adapted his views for a special government pamphlet. Critics said he watered it down due to political pressure. Koop himself later blamed "political meddlers." Some government officials and advisors, meanwhile, went so far as to try to stop the mailing altogether.

Nonetheless, in June 1988, *Understanding AIDS* was sent to every household in the U.S.

Despite all the controversy, information campaigns appeared to have an impact. Newly reported HIV infections in gay men started to decline in the late 1980s.

The number of total AIDS cases and deaths, however, continued to rise. CDC statistics in August 1987 counted 40,051 AIDS cases in the U.S. It was increasingly clear thousands, perhaps tens or hundreds of thousands, remained undiagnosed. More than 23,000 Americans had already died of the disease.

There was a long way to go until things got better.

Timeline of early historical events

circa 1931 SIVcpz virus passes to human beings in Africans and mutates into the HIV-1 virus.

1959 Earliest confirmed case of AIDS.

1978 First signs of a new contagious virus (later called HIV) and the syndrome it causes (AIDS) in the United States, Haiti, and Tanzania.

1980 Total known U.S. death toll from AIDS at thirty-one.

1981 The Centers for Disease Control reports cases of *Pneumocystis carinii* pneumonia and Kaposi's sarcoma.

1982 GRID is renamed acquired immunodeficiency syndrome, or AIDS; the same year, research identifies all the major ways the disease is transmitted.

1983 French and American researchers isolate the HIV-1 virus; Americans are warned of HIV in the blood supply.

1985 An HIV test for blood products is approved for public use.

1986 Total known U.S. deaths from AIDS top 16,000.

1987 Total known U.S. deaths from AIDS top 23,000.

1988 Surgeon General's office sends copies of *Understanding AIDS* to every U.S. household.

three
Fear, Loathing, and Change

Epidemics have a long history of creating fear and scapegoats. Panicked over plague, medieval Europeans wiped out entire Jewish communities in western and Central Europe. Nothing like that happened in the United States in the 1980s. Nor did any similar threat arise, though gays in particular faced an increased threat of individual violence and discrimination. But AIDS threw a frightening shadow on American life in the first ten years of the epidemic. Its power to create unease, even panic, didn't truly dissipate until the arrival of effective treatment in the mid-1990s.

AIDS inspired fear in large part because it was so unknown. Here was a devastating, fatal disease that had seemingly arrived out of nowhere at a time when many medical experts felt the eradication of epidemics was right around the corner.

Was AIDS caused by a virus? A bacterium? A parasite? Was it caused by certain kinds of behavior? Combinations of behaviors? Scientists at first were unsure how one person transmitted the disease to the next. Inaccurate scientific and media reports added to the panic. At one time or another, stories—some from credible sources—claimed AIDS spread by kissing, through tears, via mosquito bites, and by close (non-sexual) contact in the home.

Perhaps most frightening of all, it was impossible to tell who had AIDS because symptoms didn't appear for years.

HIV infected many kinds of people and not all of them belonged to a recognized risk group. But for most Americans, GRID—gay-related immune deficiency—said it all. HIV and AIDS became in the public mind a disease of gay white men.

Antigay feelings, like the anti-Semitism of medieval times, fed on pre-existing prejudices. A majority of Americans considered homosexuality a fringe lifestyle—repugnant, even sinful, and definitely not something they wanted to hear about on the evening news.

It's hard to imagine today, but gays as a group in the 1980s had virtually no presence in American popular culture. A talk show hosted by an openly lesbian comedian was unthinkable. On the rare occasions Hollywood or television depicted gays, it showed them as either stereotypically effeminate, or as freakish and dangerous. An actor even playing a gay character risked permanent damage to his or her career. Gay singers and musicians, with only a few exceptions, kept their sexuality to themselves.

For better or worse, the AIDS epidemic brought gay Americans more attention than they'd received at any point in history.

From the start, gays waged intense battles with political conservatives and politically active religious organizations. Both provided vital support to the administration of President Ronald Reagan. Both had a voice in setting policy, including public health policy.

Many conservatives repeatedly condemned gays as sinners. In 1983, the conservative American Family Association managed to use "perverse homosexuals," "disease carrying deviants," and "sex-crazed degenerates" in a single fundraising letter. Politicians, magazine writers, and clergyman made suggestions that the government quarantine AIDS patients, put them on watch lists, or tattoo them as HIV-positive.

Gay critics of the government's response to the epidemic didn't think it a coincidence that Reagan's administration, and the public health infrastructure it led, had failed to find HIV's cause, stop its spread, or devote what they considered the necessary funds to research these and other questions.

The gay community's frustrations weren't solely a reaction to political opponents, however. Discrimination played a real part in many gay men's lives, past and present. Until the 1970s, psychiatrists had treated homosexuality as a mental illness. Over the years the treatment for it had included electric shock, time in mental hospitals, and conversion therapy to turn them heterosexual. The American Psychiatric Association only changed its mind on the matter in 1973, and then only after pressure from gay activists.

In the 1980s, gays and lesbians could lose their job due to their sexual preference. Police didn't always investigate anti-gay violence.

To many gays, the slow advance of research and response to the AIDS crisis was more of the same thing. Except this time, they said, it was costing lives.

The fear surrounding AIDS, however, was so powerful it reverberated beyond those actually infected with the disease.

For doctors and nurses, the accidental stick with a needle was an occupational hazard. AIDS transformed it into a matter of life or death. The same seemed true of many things seen in an average emergency room every day. A bleeding accident victim, for one. A violent patient who might bite, for another.

The effects persisted outside the ER and the operating room. Officials at a Manhattan hospital told one AIDS doctor to do his laboratory work in the attic. An intern at a Worcester, Massachusetts, hospital tried to bribe colleagues to perform a minor procedure on an AIDS patient. A New York physician famous for working with HIV-infected children wasn't allowed to add a room onto his house because the people in his suburb feared he planned to open a day care center for his patients.

The stigmas wrapped around AIDS even trespassed into staffers' personal lives. "If you brought up at a dinner party [the fact] that you worked in the AIDS clinic at San Francisco General, half the room left," said one infectious disease specialist.

On more than one occasion, superiors ordered researchers to downplay and even refuse money for AIDS research. Otherwise, the institution they worked for might get the dreaded label of "AIDS hospital."

A lack of reliable information contributed to all these problems. Before 1985, the mass media covered HIV and AIDS in an on-again, off-again way, often ignoring the scientific details and the victims in favor of focusing on the bizarre and sensational, as when rumors swirled that mosquitoes transmitted the disease.

That was when the media paid attention at all. TV news took a pass on AIDS. In general, producers at the television networks decided middle America didn't care about the disease. Reporters and anchormen alike worried about describing HIV's methods of transmission in ways the audience might find offensive. And no one liked the dull video that accompanied any AIDS story. A piece on research, for instance, usually showed people in lab coats standing over test tubes. As for human interest stories, few AIDS patients wanted to be shown on TV for fear of repercussions.

Stories occasionally appeared in a big city newspaper, though rarely on the front page. *Time* and *Newsweek*, the country's two major newsmagazines, ran their first cover stories on the disease in 1983. Even in solid, straightforward coverage, though, the media focused on white, gay males. That fed the stereotype of AIDS as a gay disease and encouraged the idea it was a problem separate from the worries of most Americans.

Two stories, each shocking for different reasons, kickstarted a shift in the public's perception of the disease.

Since the 1950s, Rock Hudson had starred in every genre of Hollywood film. He was most famous for romantic comedies where he used his good looks and easygoing sense of sophistication to charm a string of leading ladies.

Hudson, fearing for his career, had kept his homosexuality from fans and close friends for decades.

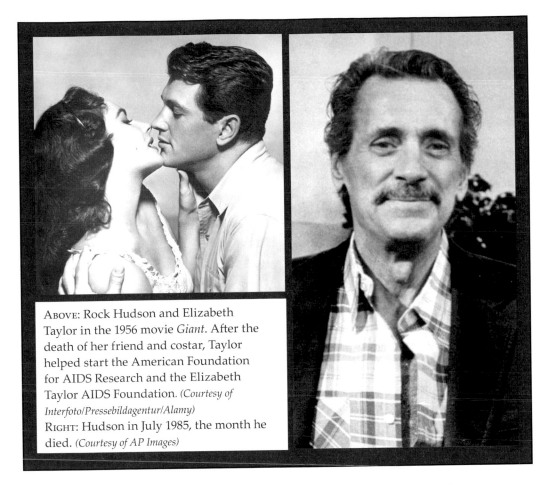

ABOVE: Rock Hudson and Elizabeth Taylor in the 1956 movie *Giant*. After the death of her friend and costar, Taylor helped start the American Foundation for AIDS Research and the Elizabeth Taylor AIDS Foundation. *(Courtesy of Interfoto/Pressebildagentur/Alamy)*
RIGHT: Hudson in July 1985, the month he died. *(Courtesy of AP Images)*

On July 15, 1985, he appeared in public after a lengthy absence. He'd lost a lot of weight. His Hollywood smile couldn't hide his sunken cheeks. Unknown to virtually anyone, he'd developed Kaposi's sarcoma.

When asked about his health, he shrugged it off as flu.

He soon flew to Paris for an experimental AIDS treatment. When he collapsed in a hotel lobby, rumors that he had the disease sparked a media frenzy.

His illness, then still unknown, led in the Sunday newspapers for July 28. Video of his July 15 appearance ran on several TV newscasts. The sight of the visibly ill Hudson, a face so familiar from the movies and television, stunned viewers. Overnight, he transformed the epidemic from statistics and grim photos of strangers to something people nationwide could relate to. He died three months after his appearance, the first—but not the last—public figure claimed by the disease.

If Hudson's death suggested anyone could get AIDS, Ryan White's story showed what could happen when an ordinary person did.

Authorities in Kokomo, Indiana, refused to allow White, a local teen diagnosed with AIDS, to attend middle school. White, a hemophiliac, had contracted AIDS from infected blood products. The local school board, pressured by fearful parents, chose to provide White with tutoring at home rather than have him in the classroom.

White's family went to court and won the right to attend school. But the teen faced harassment and insults in the classroom. Soon after, he and his family relocated to a nearby town. The story received enormous national news coverage.

To those uneducated about AIDS, White was a jarring reality check. A small-town midwesterner and a good student, White didn't conform to any stereotype of an AIDS victim. Journalists presented his story sympathetically and awakened many Americans to the fact that anyone HIV-positive, even a child, faced discrimination.

If fear of AIDS remained, the response did become more complicated. The attention paid to White and a handful of other stories similar to his, and the generally serious coverage of the disease that followed, got people talking and thinking.

If some Americans never got beyond their fear, others thought through it, aided by education or compassion or their own experiences.

By 1987, HIV and AIDS had gone mainstream. But it had been the biggest story in the gay community for six years.

Gays and lesbians provided the impetus, the volunteers, and the money for the early AIDS organizations. Only months after the initial reports on GRID, a group of gay men in New York started the Gay Men's Health Crisis, the first organization in the U.S. to provide AIDS-related services. San Francisco's gay community, the nation's largest, organized services that

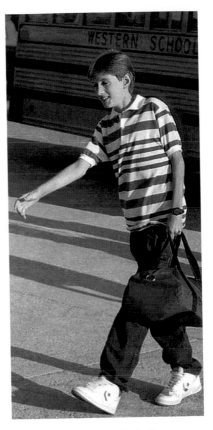

Ryan White, an AIDS victim, arriving for the first day of school after winning a court battle to attend public school in 1986. *(Courtesy of AP Images/Michael Conroy)*

ranged from hotlines to health care to serving patients too ill to travel or too poor to buy food and medicine. Boston hosted the first AIDS Walk in 1984. The idea soon spread to other cities.

Some organizations simply grew out of an individual's impulse to help. One San Francisco woman took it on herself to cook meals for, and organize delivery to, seven men with

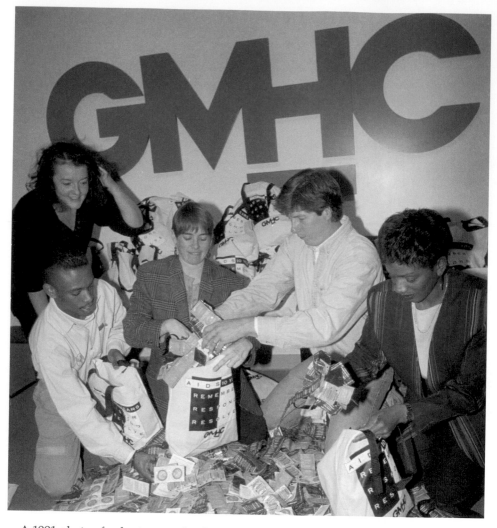

A 1991 photo of volunteers at the Gay Mens' Health Crisis loading bags with condoms, to be distributed along with leaflets promoting safe sex and AIDS awareness. (*Courtesy of Getty Images*)

AIDS. She had been inspired when she found out an AIDS-stricken neighbor had often gone without food because he was too sick to cook. In three years, her idea, called Project Open Hand, expanded to providing two meals every day for 450 people.

Counseling and companionship, even legal help, became a part of the network of services. Other groups concentrated on research into the virus, on activism to raise awareness, or on maintaining clinics and hospices. A constant lack of money limited the reach of even large organizations. But the services they provided were essential because the existing health care system had trouble coping as the epidemic expanded.

Public hospitals, supported by taxpayers and usually underfunded, dealt with huge numbers of cases, either because the patients lacked private health insurance, or because other hospitals sent them there.

The hundreds, then thousands, of AIDS patients taxed resources. AIDS differed from the usual infectious diseases. Patients didn't get better (or worse) in a short time. Government insurance like Medicare and Medicaid covered some, but never all, of the cost. The fact that some physicians wouldn't see Medicaid patients added to the load. On top of that, the medicine and machines necessary to treat their infections cost a lot of money.

Because an AIDS patient often required long-term care, he needed the kind of services more often provided by an assisted living facility or a nursing home. Existing facilities, though, were generally uncomfortable taking AIDS patients and ignorant of how to treat them. All of the facilities put together did not have the space to take everyone in need.

Meanwhile, money for AIDS had become a tug of war. AIDS advocates, especially in the gay community, demanded the Reagan administration invest more in research and education. On the other side, Reagan's supporters considered the current funding to be too generous.

In 1986, AIDS spending fell from $96 million the previous year to $85.5 million. A virologist and AIDS expert at the CDC was told, "Do as little as possible but look like you're doing a lot." Only pressure from Congress convinced the Department of Health and Human Services to shift extra money over to AIDS.

A vocal minority of activists, frustrated with government inaction, turned to demonstrations and stunts to get maximum attention. Foremost among these groups was the AIDS Coalition to Unleash Power. At times wry and outrageous, at times disruptive and insulting, ACT UP took in-your-face protest to new levels, condemning politicians as murderers, shutting down city streets, and marching on the Food and Drug Administration.

Members of ACT UP, a group of AIDS activists, protesting high AIDS drug prices in New York in 1997. *(Courtesy of AP Images/Mark Lennihan)*

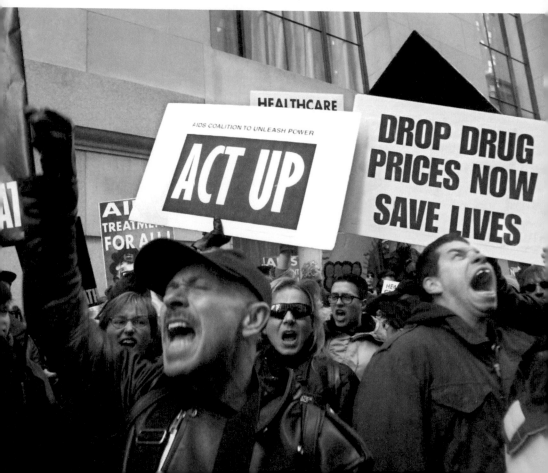

The aggressive tactics alienated many. Even within the gay community, some thought the group went too far, that the stunts did at least as much harm as good.

But some of the actions did have an effect.

AZT, the first AIDS drug, initially sold for more than $12,000 for a year's treatment, making it the most expensive drug ever released. Protests convinced the drug's manufacturer to lower it to $10,000, but activists continued to criticize the high price. On September 14, 1989, ACT UP went beyond words to express outrage to Burroughs Wellcome, AZT's maker. One member recalled:

> They didn't back down, so we upped the ante by shutting down the New York Stock Exchange, sneaking past security and using foghorns to drown out the opening bell. The company finally lowered the price three days later.

ACT UP was only part of the movement. From early on, gay groups had insisted on interaction with public health and government institutions like the CDC. Organizations staffed by articulate, educated members participated in discussions of how to react to the epidemic. Other activists raised funds from wealthy donors or lobbied politicians or administered programs.

Raising the profile of AIDS and its victims offered activists a chance to connect with the public outside the communities affected most by the disease. Connecting to the public, when it worked, created sympathy and outrage. Sympathy and outrage led Americans to pressure politicians and bureaucrats. And politicians and bureaucrats under pressure took action.

One breakthrough came with the Food and Drug Administration (FDA). Activists had wanted the FDA to speed up the approval process for new drugs. Under normal circumstances, it took an average of eight to ten years for a new medication to pass the battery of tests required for approval.

With AZT, the agency allowed patients to take the medication despite the fact it had yet to go through the years-long third stage of trials. In the end, AZT received approval in 108 days, one-seventh the usual time and by far the record for speed.

Activists cheered the FDA's new flexibility. But scientists worried. In their view, the treatments, released before proper tests were run, might have effects on health as bad as the disease. The new rules basically allowed people to experiment on themselves. From a scientific standpoint, it was impossible to study a drug's effects or whether it worked under those conditions.

AIDS patients found the attitudes ridiculous. They were dying, they said. What did an extra level of safety matter?

The FDA adopted an official accelerated approval process in 1992. New rules also allowed individuals to import experimental drugs from other countries.

In the meantime, the federal government initiated a program to help AIDS patients pay for medical and social services, and for medication. In 1990, it allocated $350 million—out of the $881 million it promised—for the new Ryan White CARE Act. (Legislators chose to honor White after he died of AIDS-related pneumonia earlier in the year.) The CARE Act became the primary source of federal money for HIV and AIDS patients.

Other new AIDS legislation included a housing program for AIDS patients and changing the Americans with Disabilities Act to prevent discrimination against people with HIV.

HIV and AIDS started to make an impact in pop culture as the 1980s ended. After Rock Hudson's death, celebrities increasingly appeared at fundraisers and fancy black-tie events against AIDS. The red ribbon became a part of the wardrobe for movie stars, activists, and everyday people alike.

In 1993, *Angels in America*, a play with AIDS-related themes, won the Pulitzer Prize for gay playwright Tony Kushner. The same year, Hollywood rolled out *Philadelphia*, the first big budget AIDS drama, with Tom Hanks and Denzel Washington in starring roles. A cable network aired a dramatization of *And the Band Played On*, an acclaimed history of the epidemic's early years.

The changing atmosphere encouraged a few famous people to admit to being HIV-positive. Greg Louganis, an Olympic gold medalist, revealed he had the disease in 1995.

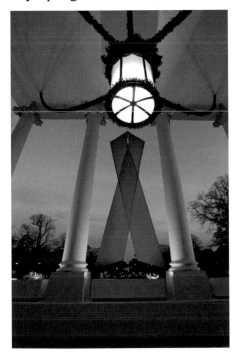

The 1991 admission and subsequent retirement of basketball star Earvin "Magic" Johnson stunned the sports world and African American community.

As the popularity of the red ribbons showed, symbols effectively called

The red ribbon has become a symbol of AIDS activism. Here, a red ribbon hangs in the north portico of the White House in observation of World AIDS Day in 2007.

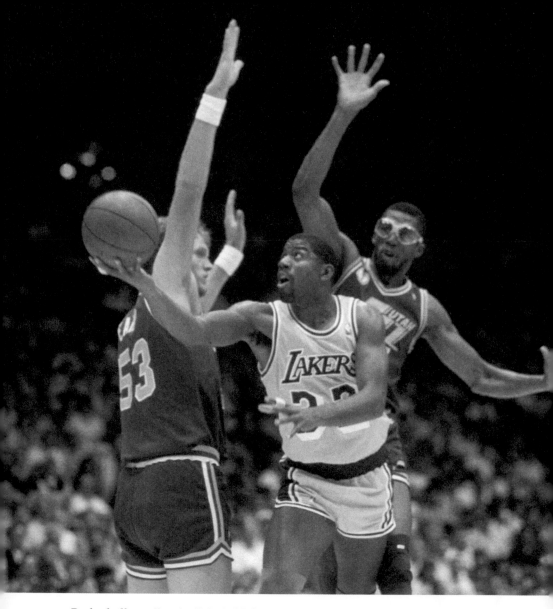

Basketball star Earvin "Magic" Johnson (center) retired from the NBA in 1991 after publicly announcing that he was infected with AIDS. *(Courtesy of AP Images/Mark Terrill)*

attention to the disease. In 1986, a San Francisco gay activist named Cleve Jones began work on the AIDS Memorial Quilt, a tapestry of three-foot-by-six-foot panels (the shape of a grave) that each represented the life of a person killed by the disease. Jones started with a friend of his.

On the weekend of October 11, 1987, a half-million people wove through and around the quilt on the National Mall in Washington, D.C. Thousands of volunteers helped display it on a twenty-city tour that raised $500,000 for AIDS charities. A documentary on the quilt and the lives it represented won an Academy Award.

For all the activism, despite the red ribbons on dresses and tuxedoes, even with more and more of the scientific community investigating every aspect of HIV, one thing remained unchanged. People continued to die.

In 1992, conditions related to AIDS killed more American men in the twenty-five to forty-four age range than any other cause. The ten-thousandth San Franciscan died the next year.

The number of cases among African Americans rose faster than the number in any other group. Latinos and women, especially African American women, also faced a greater—and growing—risk.

HIV among African Americans wasn't a new phenomenon. According to Phill Wilson, a longtime AIDS activist and educator:

> [E]ven as far back as the 80's, black gay men were disproportionately represented among gay men with H.I.V. But it was perceived as only affecting whites partly because of the way gay white men addressed the issue. They said, "forget the stigma, we're dying, and there's no time to worry about whether society likes us or not." The gay community held gay organizations accountable, gay leaders accountable, gay businesses accountable and gay media accountable. Because of this full frontal assault on the disease, AIDS became known as white and gay.
>
> When AIDS hit our community, we had so many other problems—racism, socioeconomic issues, with an overlay

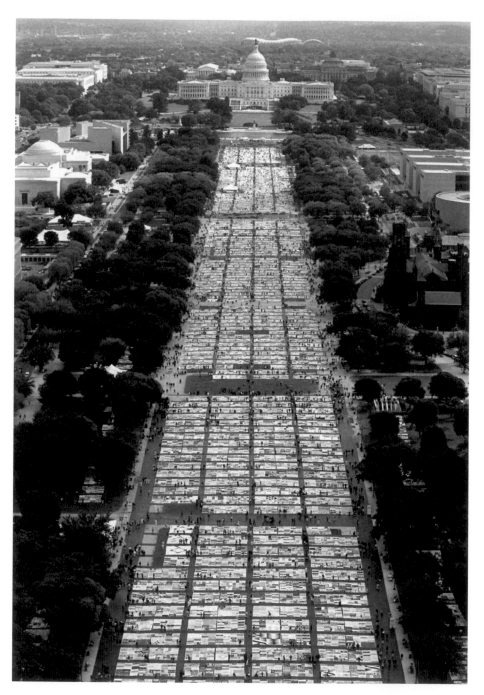

A 1996 photo of the AIDS Memorial Quilt on display between the Washington Monument and the U.S. Capitol building. *(Courtesy of AP Images/Ron Edmonds)*

of homophobia—it was easy to say, That's a white disease, not our problem. That began a conspiracy of silence around the disease.

African American attitudes toward homosexuality contributed to the silence. In fact, many blacks resisted the idea gay African Americans existed at all. Even black men who had sex with other men didn't often believe themselves to be gay. African American churches, like many white ones, wanted no part of homosexuals. This presented significant obstacles to facing down the HIV/AIDS problem because a great deal of community work in black areas orbited around churches.

Though men having sex with men remained the leading cause of infection among males, IV drug use helped the disease leap to another demographic group—minority women.

Just as drug addiction hit a disproportionate number of African Americans and Latinos, so too did HIV transmitted via needles. Drug users who caught the virus then passed it on to their sexual partners. African American women were infected more often via this route than any other group.

The increase in cases and deaths brought greater awareness of the problem, for African Americans and the country as a whole. Black political organizations and some churches began to talk openly about HIV with members.

But even in the early 2000s, AIDS activists had to strive to get community leaders to pay attention.

AIDS-related stigmas continue to contribute to HIV's spread, as well. "Whether it is a teen or a senior, folks don't take the disease seriously," said one California HIV specialist. "The taboos associated with it—promiscuity, drug usage and gay sex—make people embarrassed to admit they may be affected."

At the end of the 1980s, close to seven out of ten female HIV victims were African American or Latino. Children born to women in those groups made up the overwhelming number of HIV cases in newborns in the U.S.

In 2002, HIV killed more black women age twenty-five to thirty-four than any other cause. Two-thirds of the women reporting new HIV infections in 2005 were African American. Heterosexual contact was the leading method of transmission.

In 2005, the Centers for Disease Control reported that the AIDS rate among African Americans was ten times that of whites and almost three times that of Latinos.

When counting Americans from all racial and age groups, men are still more likely to get HIV today. But of the 1.2 million HIV-positive Americans in 2007, about one in four is a woman, with African American women far likelier to be infected than white or Latino women.

Programs and Assistance

In 2006, the U.S. government and other entities spent $1.4 billion to fund AIDS Drug Assistance Programs, or ADAPs, to help HIV-positive Americans, particularly the uninsured or those in low-income groups. The most famous is a program named for Ryan White, the teenage AIDS activist who died in 1990.

As of early 2007, about 142,000 people used the ADAPs. The majority received drugs. Thousands of others had health insurance paid for them so the expensive medication would be at least partially covered.

According to figures from June 2006, more than 70 percent of those in ADAPs had no insurance. Half lived at or below poverty level. Of all those in the programs, 54 percent had a CD4 T-cell count of below 350—not far above two hundred, the level at which HIV infection becomes AIDS.

Individual states have ADAPs as well. Who can join, the benefits allowed, and the drugs provided vary. For example, South Dakota doesn't cover protease inhibitors, while three states (Massachusetts, New Hampshire, and New Jersey) cover any prescription drug. Some programs also provide medication for some or all of the opportunistic infections recognized as related to HIV and AIDS.

four
"Slim"

HIV spread quietly in sub-Saharan Africa for decades prior to its emergence in the late 1970s. In all likelihood, the virus was on the move even when the earliest case we know of turned up in Kinshasa in 1959. Mirko Grmek, one of the first historians to investigate HIV's origins, heard that seasonal workers migrating back and forth from central Africa to South Africa in the 1950s and 1960s had suffered from sicknesses like deadly pneumonia and an unusual form of cancer suspiciously like Kaposi's sarcoma that caused purple lesions on the skin.

Starting in 1983, physicians in Tanzania treated patients suffering from a mysterious wasting disease some people in the region had nicknamed "slim." Many cases appeared in the northern towns near Lake Victoria and the Ugandan border. Locals blamed it on their tribal enemies, on traveling salesmen or witchcraft, on sex workers. The physicians were as helpless against the new disease as the traditional healers so many Tanzanians relied on for care.

The symptoms would have sounded familiar to doctors in certain parts of San Francisco and New York. People suffering from the mystery illness became weak. Purple sores appeared on the skin. Opportunistic infections attacked the lungs. Ulcers appeared on the genitals—severe, deep ulcers that resisted all treatment. Patients lost control of their bowels.

Unknown to the Tanzanians, slim had taken hold. Cases had appeared in Nairobi, the capital of Kenya. A staggering 90 percent of the women working as prostitutes in one Rwandan town were HIV-positive.

Two Tanzanian doctors, Jayo Kidenya and Klint Nyamuryekunge, and Kidenya's assistant Justhe Tkimalenka, studied the disease as it burned through the region served by their hospital. The team then sent Nyamuryekunge to present their data and medical samples at his university. His professors agreed it was something new.

Nyamuryekunge was reading scientific journals at the medical school library when he came across the early articles on AIDS in the United States. From that moment, he and his colleagues realized that they were dealing with the same disease.

The Tanzanians sent samples to the Centers for Disease Control in Atlanta. Officials there, working under the assumption that AIDS cases were concentrated in the U.S. and Haiti, were surprised to find it circulating thousands of miles away.

The CDC sent investigator Don Forthal to check into the outbreak. Forthal visited the town of Bukoba, soon to be identified as the epicenter of the Tanzanian AIDS crisis.

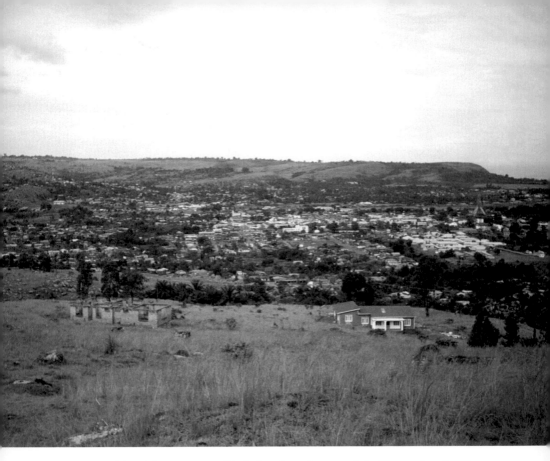

A view of the African town of Bukoba, the epicenter of the Tanzanian AIDS crisis that was first identified in 1983.

> I couldn't believe what I was seeing. In just seven days I saw maybe twenty-four or twenty-five [AIDS] patients. . . . All in this one little Bukoba hospital. These patients were so much worse off than American AIDS cases. The disease is different over there. They were just wasting away before your eyes; I could see a difference in these people in seven days' time.

Scientists had assumed AIDS would behave the same way everywhere. But affected regions in Tanzania and Uganda weren't home to the same risk groups identified in the U.S. IV drug use, for example, was nonexistent. (Reusing needles for medical procedures did exist, however.) As for gay

Africans, they lived secretively and certainly didn't organize into communities.

In Africa, HIV spread primarily through heterosexual contact. The news set off alarms among public health experts. Until then, experts thought (or hoped) that AIDS would stay within the defined risk groups. Now, it appeared that heterosexuals, the great majority of the world's population, were also theoretically at risk to catch the disease. The revelation radically changed perceptions.

HIV emerged during a time of profound change in many African societies. Like the sexual revolution in the U.S., these transformations took place on a large scale—in fact, on a far larger scale that touched virtually every aspect of African life.

One of the driving forces behind the changes was the unprecedented number of people moving from place to place.

African societies had been overwhelmingly rural since ancient times. Starting in the late 1950s, the economies of sub-Saharan Africa began to shift from the country to the city. Millions of people gave up farming to move, either temporarily or permanently, to urban areas in search of unemployment and better opportunities.

Urbanization paralleled what had happened in many Western nations in the previous two centuries. The shift took place at a tremendous rate. In the early 1960s, Nairobi had a population of 350,000. In 2007, it had jumped to an estimated 3.5 million.

The jobs attracting these millions of people included work in mining, the oil industry, various kinds of manufacturing, and the importing and exporting of goods and raw materials.

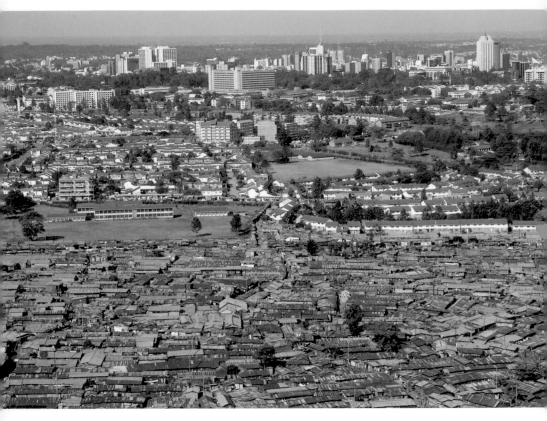

A view of Nairobi, the urban epicenter of Kenya. The urbanization of sub-Saharan African countries has increased the number of mobile workers and prostitutes, which in turn has contributed to the spread of AIDS across Africa. *(Courtesy of AP Images/ Riccardo Gangale)*

Careers related to trade, like wholesaling and selling products, were also important, as were highly mobile jobs like truck driving.

The workers on the move tended to be male and young. Many were unattached. In fact, some worked so that they could afford to get married. Regardless of marital status, a man traveled long distances, even to other countries, by himself. His wife and children, if he had a family, stayed home in the village while he worked on contract at a job that called for him to be away for months, a year, or more.

Being away from home, and making relatively good money, men had the freedom and the means to pay the sex workers in the towns and mining camps where they worked.

Sex workers represented a parallel, mobile work force, with two differences. First, they were overwhelmingly women. Second, they had few other job options. Poor, with little or no education, often considered inferior in Africa's male-dominated societies, women migrated from rural regions for many reasons—to escape a bad family situation, as refugees or orphans, or due to some other cause. But many of them found few opportunities for any kind of work, let alone a career. Untold thousands engaged in sex with multiple men, sometimes in exchange for no more than a single meal, or a canned soda, anything to keep from starving.

As in other parts of the world, multiple sex partners put the men and the sex workers at risk for sexually transmitted diseases like HIV. Often a person with the virus was unaware of the infection. Nor was their partner, nor any other partners down the line. That included other sex workers. Other customers of sex workers. Wives at home in the village.

In 1986, close to 90 percent of Nairobi's poorer prostitutes carried the virus. Similar percentages were seen in parts of Uganda and Rwanda.

But the background of HIV's spread in sub-Saharan Africa was actually more complex than men's habit of hiring sex workers.

The practice of multiple sexual partners had deep cultural roots in many parts of Africa. Where the sexual revolution in the U.S. and Europe was a rejection of tradition, promiscuity was a quite traditional part of many African cultures. People associated success with seeing multiple women. In many places, polygamy remained an option for men rich enough to afford it.

Others kept so-called "city wives," "second girlfriends," even third "wives" or "girlfriends." These women were usually not sex workers. Instead, poverty drove them to enter into semiformal relationships where they traded sex for money. Some of the city wives and second girlfriends had children or other family members to support. Others were among the untold thousands of women lacking education and unable to find a good job in Nairobi or Kinshasa or Dar es Salaam.

The same was true for the waitresses or barmaids who engaged in part-time sex work according to need or opportunity, for urban students attempting to earn living expenses or tuition, and for married women hoping to buy their freedom from a bad or abusive spouse.

While men generally considered promiscuity acceptable, a woman's view on the subject didn't matter much. African culture taught women to submit to men, come what may, and regardless of the risks. A wife protesting the presence of another woman ran the risk of violence, even divorce. Unless she had land or money, and could support herself and her family without a husband, she had little choice but to go along with whatever he did.

Many sub-Saharan nations had achieved independence from European colonizers only to find that all the country's experts were either Europeans or had fled the country. Replacing this class of people required a substantial sacrifice of time and money by governments and institutions. So did buying the equipment needed by physicians, engineers, and corporate bankers when they returned home to work. As a result, no country could afford to lose one engineer, let alone five or ten or twenty, if it had twenty.

HIV made huge inroads among this middle-class of professionals and skilled workers because they could most often afford both a wife and outside partners.

In Malawi, for example, a pregnant woman's chance of having HIV increased according to her husband's or significant other's education level. The more education, the greater the chance she was HIV-positive.

A similar link existed between HIV and professional advancement. A recent study in Zambia showed that AIDS-related illnesses killed managers at companies two-thirds of the time.

The pattern didn't hold true everywhere. But where it did, it added evidence to what shaped up as an ominous trend.

Malawian women suffering from HIV at a hospital in Malawi, Africa. *(Courtesy of Ami Vitale/Getty Images)*

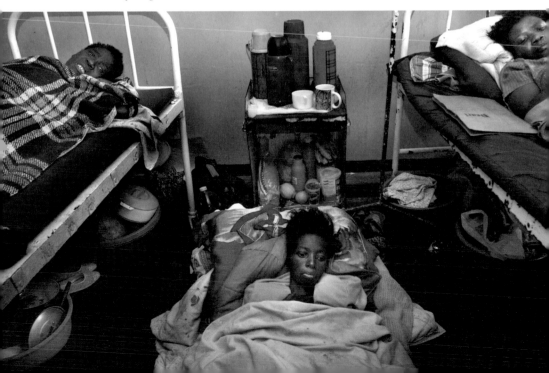

HIV killed the physicians, bankers, carpenters, bricklayers, and teachers at a chilling rate. These professionals represented a substantial—and hard-to-replace—natural resource, one vital for social and economic advancement, a reliable source of tax revenue as well as the mentors and educators for the next generation.

The effect of AIDS on ordinary workers had repercussions, too. With AIDS a growing problem in many work forces, workers became prone to call in sick to attend funerals, take care of others, or nurse their own symptoms. A study by a South African oil company found that AIDS caused a worker to miss more than twenty-seven days per year more than his or her peers. That hurt production. Furthermore, finding and training replacements cost employers money.

Meanwhile, workers in another occupation commonly associated with prosperity transmitted HIV at incredible rates.

Long-distance truck drivers were a vital part of the commercial networks transporting goods from ports to the African interior. Communities grew up along the routes where truckers sold their products and at border crossings where dozens of trucks sat for days or weeks waiting for permission to go on.

Truck drivers, like other mobile workers, engaged sex workers or visited semi-permanent girlfriends while away from home.

Researchers found they could literally trace the spread of epidemics along highways. Towns and truck stops near or on the routes had high infection rates. The numbers declined in direct relation to distance from the roads.

By 2001, more than half of South Africa's truck drivers carried the virus. AIDS had killed eighty-three of the one

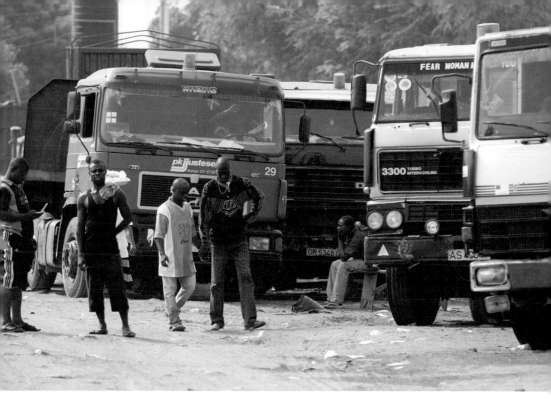

Trucks parked at a truck terminal in Tema, Ghana. Truck drivers contributed heavily to the spread of AIDS in Africa as they visited sex workers while crisscrossing the continent on trade routes. *(Courtesy of Olivier Asselin/Alamy)*

hundred drivers employed by one Malawi trucking company. The infection rate in Swaziland's truckers was twice the average of the general population.

Truck drivers faced stigmas and prejudice in some places. Elsewhere, however, towns relied on the goods the drivers hauled. Sex workers, driven by poverty, had no choice but to take them as customers. Often with unfortunate results.

With the disease becoming increasingly widespread in the 1990s, AIDS-related economic decline presented a growing threat not just to companies but to whole nations.

The fear of infection and the disease itself also added one more burden to the lives of African women.

The African epidemic struck women as hard as it did men—another difference from the early AIDS experience in the U.S. Though sex workers initially received the most attention, risk of infection also carried over to women in monogamous relationships. If a woman's husband or boyfriend wasn't monogamous, she assumed the same risk for disease that he did.

All too often, she was blamed if she became infected. Winnie Chikafumbwa, a Malawian AIDS activist, learned of that firsthand after being diagnosed as HIV-positive:

> I didn't break down until after I got home. Later in the evening when my husband came home, I broke the news to him and hell broke loose. I got the worst reaction from him. He walked out of my life that very same evening, calling me all sorts of names and blaming me that I had been unfaithful to him and that I was a prostitute. He left me with four children under my care and went to stay with another woman, and thus infected that other woman, too, because I later learned that he had already been tested and found HIV positive but could not gather courage to tell me.

AIDS also spread among young, unmarried women. In much of sub-Saharan Africa, girls generally became sexually active earlier than boys. More significantly, their first partners were generally older men rather than people their own age. These older partners might be authority figures or married men with money looking for a "city girlfriend." Since they had several past and even current partners, these men had greater odds of exposure to HIV. And, of course, greater odds of passing it on to young women.

As a result, African women caught HIV on average five or ten years earlier than men. In one Ugandan town, for example, teenage girls were twenty times as likely as male peers to be HIV-positive. Compared to men in their late teens, twice as many women in Malawi had HIV.

The discovery of human immunodeficiency virus and the development of the blood test to detect it gave researchers a tool to uncover the extent of the disease's spread. Statistics suggested an epidemic with hundreds of thousands, if not millions, of infected Africans. At the time the disease appeared unstoppable in the U.S. What chance did the impoverished nations of sub-Saharan Africa have against it?

African governments, in fact, had a hard time admitting to AIDS at all, let alone an AIDS crisis.

Different governments had different reasons for their response, or lack of response. Dictators or hyper-nationalistic patriots led a number of countries. Out of pride or arrogance, they couldn't admit such a problem had developed under their leadership.

Other countries had to weigh the reaction from neighbors and the world at large, especially the economic impact. Just the word "AIDS" provoked strong and often irrational feelings. Another country might refuse to buy goods for fear of somehow importing the virus. Reports of an out-of-control AIDS epidemic would certainly scare away desperately needed tourists.

Resistance had other causes, as well. In the 1980s, many Africans refused to believe the idea (then unproven) that HIV originated on their continent. Politicians and patriots alike condemned the idea as racism or an attempt to pin the AIDS tragedy on Africa.

Research linking the disease to chimpanzees reinforced the sensitivity about racism. To many Africans, this sounded very much like the old notion that blacks were closer to animals than to white Europeans.

At the same time, African scientists on the front lines dealt with professional disrespect, adding to the overall bad feelings. More than once, Western scientists jetted into an African country for a week or two, used local experts for their connections and data, and then returned to the U.S. or Europe to reap reward from the findings—elbowing out their African colleagues in the process.

Some countries did recognize the threat. But circumstances, and above all poverty, prevented an effective response. In huge parts of sub-Saharan Africa, AIDS was one of a long list of problems. Ordinary people often didn't have adequate clothes, sufficient food or fresh water, proper shelter, or safe sanitation.

Under those conditions, medical care was a luxury. The average Ugandan spent a single dollar—$1—on medical care in a year. Overall, sub-Saharan Africa's medical systems, inadequate even before AIDS arrived, had no chance against the epidemic.

A hospital ward on the AIDS-ridden Uganda-Tanzania border was a room with antique steel-framed beds and unwashed mattresses. If the beds were full, a patient slept on the floor. Even the most committed doctor could only watch as his patients wasted away. In an average day he might deal with nurses terrified to touch the patients, with electrical power that only came on for part of the day, with the fact the hospital's desperately needed supplies might be stolen en route from the capital, with government pressure to falsify medical records to hide AIDS cases, with HIV-contaminated blood, with needles that had to be inadequately sterilized and reused because they had no others.

Clinics in the villages dealt with even worse conditions and seldom had a trained physician on staff.

Uganda organized one of the first campaigns to fight back against HIV. Conceding that Ugandan men wouldn't give up polygamy or promiscuity, the government tried to convince men to stay within their chosen system of wives and girl-friends, and avoid casual sex with prostitutes, co-workers,

Loveth Okundaye (left) speaks to a resident outside a mobile counseling clinic in southern Nigeria. Okundaye councils truck drivers and prostitutes to raise awareness about AIDS. *(Courtesy of Emmanuel Goujon/AFP/Getty Images)*

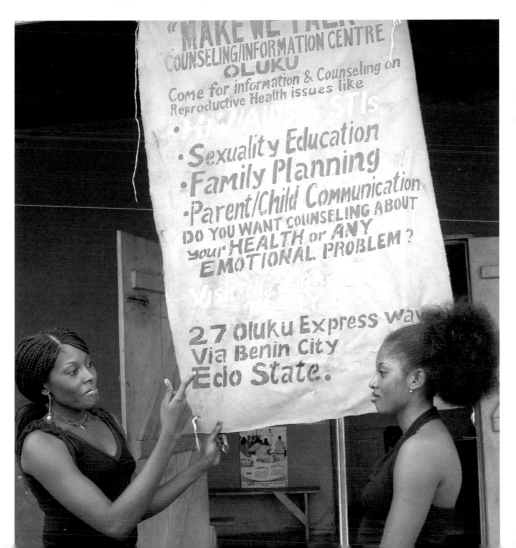

students, and church congregants—all of whom were popular short-term partners.

The campaign appeared to have some success. Infection rates for slim did fall. In the early 1990s, Uganda added safe sex campaigns that promoted condom use. Surveys indicated that casual sexual activity returned to its old levels. Yet HIV rates failed to rise.

Anti-AIDS campaigns in other countries, however, had mixed results. Conservative Christians and Muslims refused to go along, preferring to promote abstinence. Africans in general didn't want to hear about AIDS—that disease of other people—any more than the average American. Safe-sex messages failed to find listeners even when inexpensive or free condoms became available.

Women's weak position in society left them with few options if a partner refused safe sex. Even if willing to stand up for herself, she normally didn't have legal protection against a violent husband or boyfriend. Police generally agreed with the idea that a man had a free hand with "his" woman.

Campaigns of all kinds also ran up against a lack of education. Illiteracy was widespread, especially among women. Even people able to read and write in one or more languages sometimes worked in countries where the native language was unknown to them.

At the end of 1995, North America reported a total of 1,281,000 HIV infections (people both living and deceased). Western Europe's cases stood at 838,000 and Oceania, with Australia and New Zealand, at 32,000. That added up to around 2.2 million.

Sub-Saharan Africa, by contrast, had a total of 19.2 million cases. Each day, about 5,000 people became infected.

Nearly 80 percent of the world's fatal AIDS cases came from the region—twice as many victims as in the rest of the world combined and more than one hundred times as many victims as in North America. Just over 56 percent were women.

Throughout the 1990s, Africa's epidemic increasingly became a catastrophe targeting people in the fifteen-to-twenty-nine age bracket. This fit with a pattern seen around the world. Epidemics often emerged in a spurt of sudden growth over a period of a few years. During that period—a phase researchers called saturation—the virus infected the bulk of individuals most at risk.

During the next phase, new cases appeared more and more in young adults as they became sexually active.

Those infected with HIV weren't the disease's only victims, however. There were also the survivors, the AIDS orphans.

According to the United Nations Children's Fund (UNICEF), AIDS-related conditions had killed both parents of about 5.1 million children in 2005. The number of families where one parent had died was far higher.

Children typically ended up with the mother when the father died. If the extended family agreed to help, the orphaned children had a safety net to provide for emotional and physical needs. But that was a big if. The stigma surrounding AIDS was strong. A dead man's family might blame an innocent mother—as Winnie Chikafumbwa's husband had blamed her—and drive her and her children away.

AIDS dismantled traditions that had endured for generations. Among Kenya's Luo community, a dead man's brother took the widow as one of his wives. Though not always agreeable to the woman, the situation at least guaranteed protection

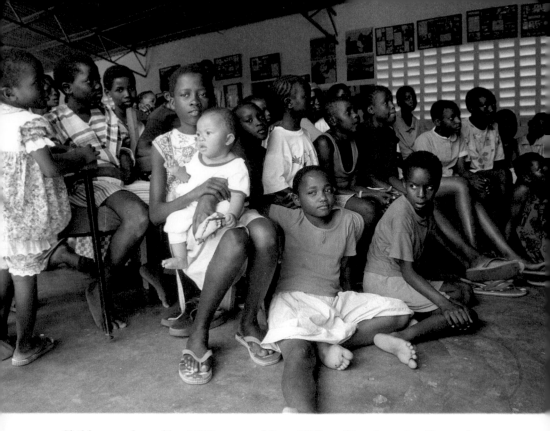

Children orphaned by AIDS, many of them HIV positive also, attending a class at a children's home in Kenya. *(Courtesy of AP Images/Khalil Senosi)*

for her and her children, and women often went along with the custom.

When the recently widowed Milka Achieng found out she had HIV, her in-laws "behaved angrily and told me I could not stay there as I would only bring them another coffin. One day I went to town and when I returned they had removed the sheet-metal roofing. They beat me and chased me away."

Achieng was left destitute, living in a nearby slum with her three children.

The loss of a parent, devastating enough, was often just the start. Because many Africans considered AIDS so shameful, they looked down on the children of victims. Orphans in many parts of Africa faced prejudice, despite having nothing to do with their parent's illness, despite being free of HIV themselves. Neighbors shunned them at church and school, relatives ignored them, and communities isolated them or drove them away. This added to the depression that followed a parent's death and to the sense of shame felt by the child. In regions where medical resources were few, orphans had no access to psychological help to deal with the intense emotional traumas.

Without a doubt, many Africans took in orphans out of love, compassion, or tradition. But even in a good situation, a new child or children added to a family's financial stress, since the orphans had to be fed, clothed, and sent to school. The need for money sometimes forced children to leave school to make money through work (often under terrible conditions), prostitution, or begging. If a choice had to be made between children, girls—considered less important—were usually pulled out of the classroom instead of boys.

A tradition of caring for abandoned children spurred many communities to action. But efforts to provide basic needs like blankets and food were often overwhelmed by the number of orphans.

Said Stephen Lewis, the UN Special Envoy for HIV-AIDS in Africa from 2001 to 2006, "The policies for orphans, more often than not, are a grab bag of frantic interventions, where faith-based and community-based groups try desperately to cope with the numbers, but rarely have either the capacity or the resources."

AIDS orphans were especially vulnerable to exploitation. Research found an increased threat of abuse. Relatives or others used them as labor. Members of the extended family seized their parents' property for themselves.

The phrase "AIDS orphan" became a negative label. African governments and media often portrayed these children as a future threat to society destined to end up as child soldiers or criminals. Studies found little evidence to support this image. But it persisted and remains strong today.

As of 2005, South Africa had the most children orphaned by AIDS. The United Nations estimated that 1.2 million AIDS orphans lived in the country, with the number expected to reach 2 million in 2010.

According to the UN, an estimated 20 million children will have lost one or both parents to AIDS in sub-Saharan Africa by 2010.

The region's future with the disease may be just as grim. A combination of forces—mobility, economics, culture, poverty—have contributed to mind-boggling levels of infection.

In Lesotho and Zimbabwe, HIV infects one out of three adults.

More than 10 percent of all the HIV-positive people in the world live in South Africa.

In Swaziland in 2003, almost 39 percent of all adults carried the virus. Because of AIDS, the average Swazi male can only expect to live to age thirty-two.

Poor, lacking much of a health care infrastructure, sub-Saharan Africa still trails far behind the Western world when it comes to treating HIV and AIDS. That would be true if nothing had changed since 1981.

But, as it turned out, things had changed.

Another Mobile Occupation

Soldiers and disease have gone hand in hand since ancient times. Whether it's packing men into ships or trucks, or marching them into other countries, or subjecting them to months of filth and stress and bad food, war is an excellent setting for disease.

Africa saw a lot of wars in the years after World War II. The men fought as armies, as militias, as lawless forces with no particular cause. Many of these conflicts forced huge numbers of people to move to new places—not in search of jobs, but because they were refugees.

The Lake Victoria region was notably unstable. Uganda's dictator of the 1970s, Idi Amin, unleashed years of exile, mass murder, and refugee flight. His policies disrupted trade so much that the Ugandan economy disappeared. Smuggling goods across the Tanzanian border or by boat over Lake Victoria became the primary economic activity. Semi-lawless camps and towns sprang up to serve the illegal trade.

Whether or not the violence and instability of the era encouraged HIV's spread is open to argument. But the first wave of outbreaks struck soldiers especially hard. Eighty percent of military personnel in some parts of Uganda carried HIV. Even today, military recruits are at higher-than-average risk for infection across sub-Saharan Africa.

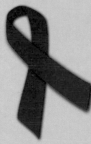

The Treatment Revolution

O ne of most terrifying aspects of the early AIDS epidemic was the fact that nothing worked against the disease. No medicine stopped it, certainly none cured it, and no vaccine prevented it. The lack of options created an atmosphere in which desperate patients were willing to try anything—in essence, experimenting on their own bodies. A long line of fakes and con artists appeared, supplemented here and there by an honest scientist who let compassion override caution, to provide miracle cures. Some of these "cures" were a challenge to good sense and dignity, many were expensive, and all were worthless.

But epidemics have always inspired bizarre remedies based in folk medicine and superstition, in faith, in inaccurate or wrong-headed science, in the faintest kind of hope.

The ancient Romans wrote *abracadabra* on strips of papyrus to guard against malaria. Renaissance-era Europeans dying of syphilis used a mercury cure that, though ineffective against the disease, did cause their hair and teeth to fall out. Newspapers in 1918 carried ads for syrups and other concoctions that supposedly treated fatal influenza.

AIDS added to this sad and lengthy tradition.

A Mexican drug called isoprinosine was still in the testing stage in the U.S. when it came to the attention of American AIDS patients. It sounded so promising that one activist organization wrote a how-to guide on sneaking it past border agents. Isoprinosine didn't work.

AL-721 was an Israeli product that used egg whites and had shown promise during early stages of research. It didn't work, either.

For $15,000 and airfare, a patient could fly to a Caribbean island to be treated with salt water charged with electricity.

A company based in a Miami Beach mall marketed reticulose, an allegedly surefire cure that took three weeks and $6,000.

Another dubious treatment took blood from a patient, added ozone to it, and returned it to the body.

Physician Henry Heimlich, inventor of the Heimlich maneuver, pitched one of the more high-profile treatments. Heimlich treated AIDS by infecting a patient with malaria. After the malarial fever burned a few weeks, Heimlich cured the malaria with medication. Heimlich insisted the process would get rid of both malaria and HIV. Using a gift for fundraising, he convinced celebrities to donate hundreds of thousands of dollars toward a treatment clinic in Mexico, away from the reach of American regulations. When things didn't work out, the clinic relocated farther away, to China.

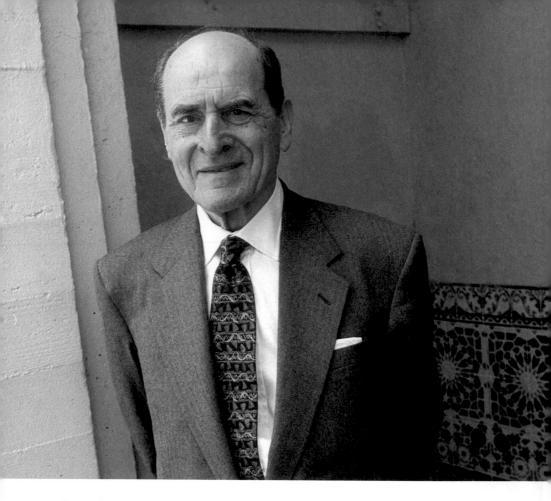

Some physicians and activists criticized Henry Heimlich (above) for profiting from a discredited "cure" for AIDS during the epidemic's early years. *(Courtesy of Dan Callister/Getty Images)*

Holistic medicine stores sold products said to help boost the immune system. Goat milk supposedly affected the virus. Taking huge amounts of vitamins was another, more popular treatment. While herbs and vitamins might have helped with nutrition, and while HIV patients benefited from good nutrition, such products did nothing to stop the virus or delay the onset of AIDS.

Not all of the treatments were the work of frauds. Serious researchers looked at some of the drugs, including isoprinosine.

These products actually fell under the heading of experimental treatment.

The first truly useful medications didn't treat the disease itself but instead worked against AIDS-related opportunistic infections. Antibiotics, for example, helped knocked down some conditions caused by bacteria. But even these old healing tools had limits.

The first glimpse of hope appeared with a drug shelved years before. Azidothymidine, or AZT, was an old and ineffective leukemia drug. Tests showed it slowed down the destruction of the important CD4+ T-cells in advanced AIDS cases. The pharmaceutical company Burroughs Wellcome

AZT was one of the first drugs to show signs of stopping the AIDS virus from destroying T-cells. *(Courtesy of National Cancer Institute)*

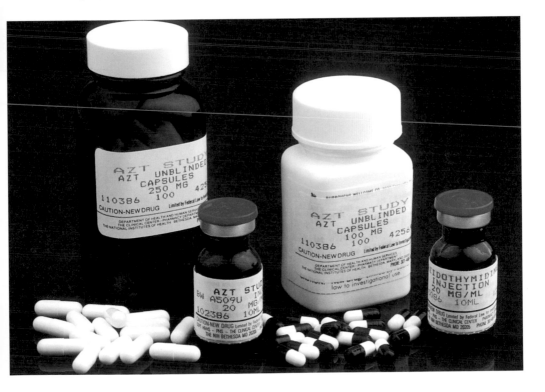

patented AZT in 1986. The Food and Drug Administration okayed it on March 20 of the following year.

"Today's approval marks an important step, but by no means a final victory, in our ongoing war against AIDS," said Robert E. Windom, assistant secretary for health at the Department of Health and Human Services. "[AZT] is not a cure for AIDS, but it has a demonstrated ability to improve the short-term survival of AIDS patients. . . . [T]oday's action means that significant medical relief will be available to thousands of those afflicted with this dreaded disease."

AZT had limits. Its efficiency faded the more it was used. A patient gained, on average, just an extra year to live. The cost was also high—$1.80 per pill, or around $10,000 per year. Under pressure from activist groups, Burroughs Wellcome cut the price by 20 percent on two different occasions.

AZT's side effects were also a serious problem. Patients suffered severe cramps, headaches, fever, nausea, bone marrow damage, extreme weight loss, and other symptoms.

"I never quit throwing up for a year," said one woman in 1997. "It was like morning sickness twenty-four hours a day. It was a horrible year."

Unfortunately, nothing else existed. Nonetheless, there were patients who chose to stop taking AZT rather than live their last months in agony.

Despite its shortcomings, AZT changed attitudes about the disease. Once considered invincible, and a death sentence for its victims, AIDS suddenly seemed closer to becoming a treatable, if lifelong, illness. If this first treatment had limits, it still gave people hope there would be a second and third and fourth treatment, each safer and more effective than its predecessors. Cures and vaccines sounded possible again.

AZT continued to be the main treatment option into the early and mid-1990s. In 1994, the government approved a new, short-term use. When administered to mothers and to their babies shortly after birth, AZT cut the chance of HIV being transmitted to the child. This cut cases of infants with HIV to almost zero in the U.S. and raised hopes of doing the same in Africa.

Around the same time, more new drugs appeared to deal with AIDS-related infections. From 1991 to 1993, the FDA either approved or allowed early, pre-approval use of medicine to treat *pneumocystis carinii* pneumonia, one of the more familiar life-threatening conditions in advanced AIDS cases, and certain cytomegalovirus infections.

The agency also okayed the use of existing drugs for extreme weight loss and fungal infections common to AIDS patients.

During the same period, researchers discovered that mixing AZT with certain other drugs produced a potent drug cocktail. In some patients, the cocktail got better results than AZT alone. It also partially foiled HIV's nasty habit of evolving into forms that made AZT less effective, a concept known as drug resistance.

Of the drug combinations under scrutiny, one of the most promising involved a new medication called a protease inhibitor.

A protease inhibitor worked by blocking one of the virus's essential functions. When buds of HIV began to break out of an infected cell, an enzyme known as the protease splits the virus's proteins into various parts. This process is necessary for HIV to mature into an active agent and move on to infect new cells.

Protease inhibitors, as the name suggests, prevented the protease from doing its work. The budding copies of HIV never reached maturity and couldn't infect new cells.

For all its promise, a protease inhibitor had one serious drawback from a biological point of view. When taken alone, the drug encouraged HIV to evolve into mutant strains able to resist the drug's effects. Scientists then discovered that combining it with other medications both offset the problem and helped all the drugs work better.

To win against HIV required a drug that not only knocked down the virus, but knocked it down so fast it had no chance to mutate into new, drug resistant forms. The idea was to hit HIV from three directions.

Ingredient one was AZT or one of the handful of AZT substitutes.

Ingredient two was a drug that short-circuited HIV's ability to convert its genetic material into DNA.

Ingredient three, the protease inhibitor, took care of the strains of virus that escaped ingredients one and two.

The three-pronged attack, called combination therapy, revolutionized treatment for HIV and AIDS. Work by David Ho, one of the world's leading AIDS researchers, had helped lead to the new treatment. Ho had proven that HIV reproduced itself in huge amounts from the start of the initial infection. The idea contradicted the prevailing thought that, once inside the body, HIV worked very slowly. As Ho and his collaborators showed, HIV spent the years of the asymptomatic phase infecting cells and, significantly, mutating into new strains.

The results, as Ho noted, were miraculous:

> For the first time we see some deathly ill patients totally recover after two to three weeks of good therapy, and we

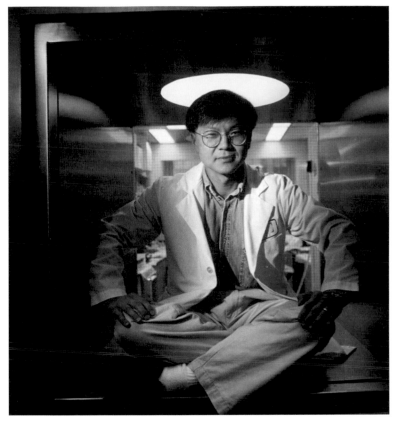

A 1996 photo of David Ho, one of the world's leading AIDS researchers.

had within our own clinical studies several patients who had essentially no CD4 T-cells left and were thin, wasted, no longer very functional, and some even bedridden. To have those cases return gradually over a few weeks or a couple of months to a state where they would return to work is certainly impressive. So this in the field has been termed the Lazarus syndrome by some folks, and that is true; there are a number of such examples where people got out of their deathbed after a few weeks of therapy.

Physicians didn't delay getting the drug cocktail to AIDS patients. Tens of thousands of people started on the regimen in 1996. For some, the body began to again produce healthy CD4+ T-cells. Levels of the virus dropped dramatically, in fact so low that blood tests no longer detected HIV.

Physicians and scientists noted immediate results. In 1997, deaths from AIDS in the U.S. fell 47 percent, from 31,130 the previous year to approximately 16,700.

With so many patients on combination therapy, the problems related to it soon became apparent. Just keeping up with the pills overwhelmed some people. The drug cocktail required a patient to take thirty pills or other forms of medicine every day, some with meals, some with fatty food, some on an empty stomach, and at all hours.

Missing a certain number of doses—easy to do with the amount of medication involved—allowed HIV to roar back. It also accelerated the virus's evolution into drug-resistant forms.

Drug resistance, in fact, was an issue for all patients, even those able to keep up with the regimen. In some people, the virus reappeared in blood tests a year or more into what had seemed like successful therapy.

The virus, wily as always, hid in macrophages (white blood cells responsible for "eating" invading microbes) and in a small percentage of the CD4+ T-cells, where a particle of HIV then turned itself off and waited for the opportunity to reproduce. Medicine could not reach these virus particles, didn't even recognize them as virus particles.

For some people, then, the drugs promised new life and suddenly failed them.

Overenthusiastic press reports often played up the miracle of combination therapy without detailing the drawbacks. The drugs, though truly a breakthrough, didn't cure HIV. A person with the virus could still transmit it, no matter how good they felt, and regardless of whether it showed up in their blood. The fact that thousands of people continued to contract HIV over the next ten years showed that reports of the disease's defeat were premature.

Side effects occurred, as with earlier treatments. Combination therapy brought on serious conditions like diabetes, inflammation of the pancreas, and abnormally low numbers of red blood cells. Protease inhibitors sometimes caused a patient's mouth or hands and feet to go numb. Skin conditions—rashes, sensitivity to touch—were an issue, as were intense cases of herpes. Dehydration and kidney stones taxed the kidneys. Many patients complained of uncontrollable diarrhea that came on without warning.

The protease inhibitors also caused body fat to collect behind the shoulders, in the neck or stomach, or in the breasts. At the same time, the face and limbs became leaner, contributing to a sickly appearance.

Side effects caused missed doses or convinced patients to give up on combination therapy altogether. Unfortunately, partial or short-lived treatments also created drug resistance. Some scientists worried that half-hearted drug use would create an HIV super-bug able to survive the existing medications.

Even those with a fatal illness had a limit. Few people could keep up with taking daily handfuls of drugs or dealing with side effects for the rest of their lives. The drug resistance danger made it even more important to make combination therapy not only more effective but easier (fewer pills, for instance) and more bearable (fewer side effects).

All of the problems, all of the trial-and-error involved in finding the right drugs and the right doses, created frustrations for both patients and physicians. But the more farsighted doctors and scientists had expected setbacks. AIDS medicines had been on a fast track for approval and bypassed the years-long drug trials. In the past, problems with dosages and side effects had showed up in test subjects, and were worked out by research, before the drugs became available to the public. Now, in essence, all HIV/AIDS patients were the test subjects.

Research turned to creating a second generation of medications both more user-friendly and able to step in when drug resistance pushed the first generation aside.

In the meantime, an HIV-positive patient faced the high cost of the life-saving treatment. Combination therapy involved more than drugs. It required laboratory tests to check on virus levels and CD4+ counts and additional treatment to handle side effects. In all, a year of combination therapy could cost $20,000 or more.

Patients with health insurance often coped (though it varied). Medicaid payments in states with more generous programs, like California, helped those who qualified. But the unemployed, or those working at a job without health benefits, had a harder time, especially since Medicaid, a program aimed at poor Americans, often was closed to them. Federal and state programs picked up some of the slack, but not nearly all of it.

If some Americans had trouble with the cost, few people in the developing world had a chance of getting treatment. At the end of the 1990s, this became a leading cause for AIDS activists, both in Africa and the West.

By the year 2000, the number of South Africans carrying HIV had already surpassed that of every country in Africa. The figure at the end of 2005 stood at 5.5 million, the highest in the world. Among sexually active women the rate was

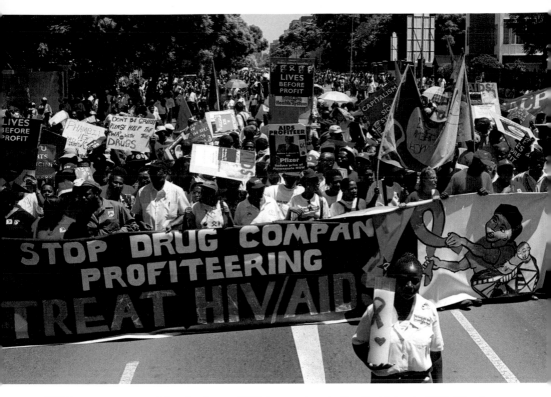

AIDS protesters marching for lower HIV drug prices in South Africa in 2001. *(Courtesy of AP Images/Christian Schwetz)*

one in four. Only one other African country, Nigeria, carried more than 2 million cases.

An epidemic raged despite the fact that the country had the continent's best medical system. To some degree, however, health care still reflected the apartheid system that defined South African life until the 1990s. Whites were overall wealthier than blacks and lived in areas with better hospitals and care. Though the medical system had started to deliver somewhat better for middle-class and professional blacks, the great majority of the black population was poor and lacked good health care.

South Africa's then-president, Thabo Mbeki, added to the problem. Shortly after assuming office in 1999, Mbeki outraged the world scientific community by questioning whether HIV was the sole cause of AIDS. While willing (at times) to admit HIV played a role, he insisted poverty, malnutrition, and other factors were also involved and perhaps even more important.

Mbeki's government didn't outlaw AIDS drugs. But the public health system refused to provide them. When pressured to buy cheap generic substitutes for the medications, the government still said no, insisting that doing so would mean trade problems with the United States.

The claim had some truth to it.

The administration of President Bill Clinton opposed plans to import generic drugs for AIDS or any other disease.

South African president Thabo Mbeki speaks to AIDS experts in 2000. *(Courtesy of AP Images)*

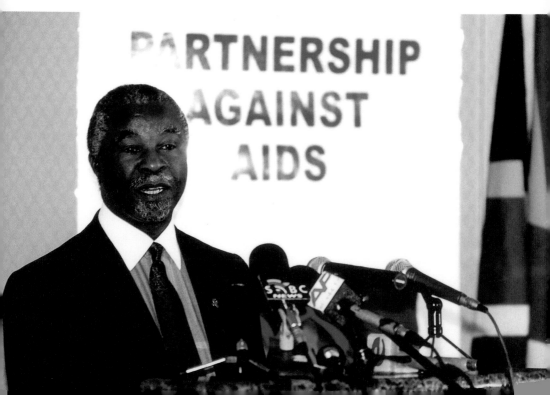

Under Clinton, the U.S. government agreed with drug company arguments that knockoff generics trespassed on their patents and that patents, like all intellectual property, had to be protected. Without protection, they said, companies had no incentive to research and develop new drugs, since generics would undercut any chance of making a profit.

Different countries dealt with the patent issue in different ways. India, for instance, simply ignored patent laws. Several Indian companies made generic copies of AIDS drugs (and many others) that cost a fraction of American medicines. These generics were sold throughout the developing world. (Laws prevented them from being brought into the U.S.)

There was also the option of a compulsory license. In the event of a health emergency, international agreements allowed poor nations to legally go around patents held by drug compa-

Technicians work at an Indian pharmaceutical company that manufactures inexpensive, generic AIDS drugs. *(Courtesy of Jean-Marc Giboux/Getty Images)*

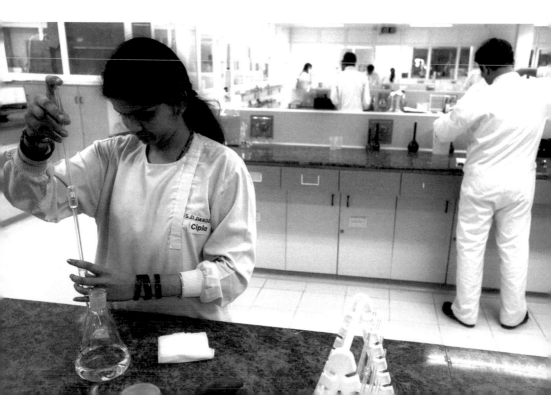

nies. A country issued a compulsory license to manufacturers to make generic knockoffs of drugs useful in dealing with the emergency. The license also allowed a nation to import generic drugs from abroad.

The Clinton administration, however, threatened to use trade sanctions to punish South Africa if it approved the manufacture or import of generics. To highlight the issue's importance, Vice President Al Gore personally led the effort to warn off the Mbeki government.

While the threats had an effect, far more than international pressure was at work. Mbeki refused to get behind the distribution of AIDS medicines even when conflict with the U.S. wasn't an issue.

Public health officials sympathetic to Mbeki proved unwilling to provide AZT to both AIDS patients and HIV-positive pregnant women. When a drug manufacturer offered to give away nevirapine, a cheaper alternative to AZT used to prevent HIV crossing over from mothers to newborns, the government still dragged its feet. Its program to pass out nevirapine reached only about 10 percent of new mothers.

A lawsuit by South African AIDS activists led to a court order to expand the program. But the Mbeki administration appealed, delaying things further.

Manto Tshabalala-Msimang, the minister of health, promoted garlic, lemon, and African potatoes as immune boosters instead.

Mbeki and members of his government attracted more criticism by dismissing AIDS drugs as a plot to poison black Africans, as toxins that Western drugs companies wanted to test using Africans as guinea pigs. The knowledge that the white apartheid government had once looked into biological weapons against blacks added fuel to the conspiracy theories.

Drug companies did sometimes cut prices for the African market. Yet even slashing a year's worth of medication to $1,000 (compared to, say, $20,000-plus in the U.S.) meant little. The average AIDS victim in sub-Saharan African was as far from paying $1,000 per year as she was from paying $10,000 or $20,000. Even in relatively wealthy South Africa, the average yearly income was around $2,600. In most of sub-Saharan Africa, it was far less.

Furthermore, the Indian generic versions of the same drugs cost less than $700. The $300 difference between the American and Indian price was an enormous savings considering the government bought for tens of thousands of patients.

Mbeki eventually okayed the import of generics when the Clinton administration, and later the government of George W. Bush, eased the pressure.

But the country's plans still faced opposition from drug manufacturers. Thirty-nine pharmaceutical companies sued to prohibit South Africa from manufacturing generic AIDS drugs or importing them from abroad.

The lawsuit led to a public relations disaster. People around the world condemned the action. Even a late effort to cut prices further failed to generate goodwill. With the European Union, World Health Organization (WHO), Doctors Without Borders, and other organizations on South Africa's side, and with the drug industry's reputation taking a huge hit, the companies dropped the suit in 2001. In turn, South African officials agreed to rewrite some of the country's regulations.

The battleground over cost stretched beyond Africa.

Brazil, like South Africa, entered the twenty-first century with a serious AIDS problem and conflict with the U.S. and pharmaceutical companies. The Brazilians used raw materials from India to manufacture generics, including knockoffs of protease inhibitors. As result, prices for AIDS drugs in Brazil fell 70 percent. The public health system saved more than $600 million.

But other developing world nations hesitated to start manufacturing their own generics, because it was too expensive to start up the factories, or for fear of U.S. retaliation, or both.

The Brazilians continued to battle with pharmaceutical corporations into 2007. For years, the government negotiated over Efavirenz, a drug manufactured by Merck. Merck eventually agreed to sell the drug at $1.10 per pill, down from the original cost of about $1.59.

But Merck had already lowered the price in Thailand to about sixty-five cents per pill. Brazil wanted the same discount. Merck refused to go lower. Brazil refused to pay.

In May of 2007, President Luiz Inacio Lula da Silva invoked the country's right to issue a compulsory license. That cleared the way to import a generic version of Efavirenz made in India. The compulsory license, officials said, would save the country almost $237 million over five years.

Drug company executives replied that such tactics threatened to curb further research and innovation. Patients and activists in the U.S., sometimes backed by physicians, clashed with manufacturers as well.

In 2004, an organization of doctors and other health care providers protested when Abbott Laboratories raised the price of Norvir from $50 to $250 for a month's supply. Norvir was an important drug. In addition to being a protease inhibitor, it kept the other drugs in combination therapy from being absorbed quickly. Because the drugs remained in the bloodstream longer, they worked better. Norvir was also in Kaletra, a popular Abbott drug that mixed it with another protease inhibitor.

Doctors in Boston, Los Angeles, and elsewhere boycotted Abbott drugs and threatened to not take part in drug studies with the company. Abbott countered that the new price corresponded to Norvir's importance and that it took money to fund further research.

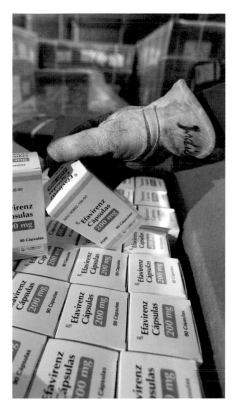

A Brazilian customs worker shows boxes of the generic HIV medicine Efavirenz. The Brazilian government bought the medicine, made by a pharmaceutical company in India, through UNICEF. *(Courtesy of AP Images)*

The disputes continue. In early 2007, the Swiss pharmaceutical company Novartis filed a lawsuit to prevent Indian companies from making generic copies of a cancer drug. AIDS advocates worried that a Novartis victory in the case would also allow Western drug manufacturers to block generic versions of important AIDS drugs. That could have far-reaching effects. Up to 80 percent of the AIDS medicine used in developing countries comes from India.

In the meantime, researchers have kept searching for ways to make taking the drugs easier. The number of pills involved, and the demanding schedule for taking them, raised one of the biggest obstacles to patients getting the most benefit from the medication.

In July 2006, the FDA approved Atripla, a medication that contained three of the most recommended drugs (though not a protease inhibitor). With Atripla, patients took a single pill one time per day, a far cry from the handfuls of pills needed ten years earlier.

Andrew von Eschenbach, the acting commissioner of the FDA, called it "a landmark for those suffering with HIV and AIDS. . . . [C]ompliance with therapy is as important as the therapy itself for a successful outcome."

The new pill represented breakthroughs in another area, too. It came about through an unusual alliance between Gilead Sciences and Bristol-Myers Squibb, two competing pharmaceutical companies. Each owns the rights to at least one of the drugs in Atripla. The cooperation between two rival manufacturers raised hopes for future innovations in treatment.

The Bush administration planned to look at the drug as part of its $15 billion program to treat HIV and AIDS in Africa. Pills sold in the U.S. (at full price) were salmon-colored. Those intended for sale (at reduced price) in the developing world were white. Manufacturers continued to research how to add a protease inhibitor to Atripla to further simplify treatment.

As it stands, though, no one is sure how long the current medications will work. "We are still in the infancy of antiviral treatment for HIV and AIDS," said Luc Montagnier, the co-discoverer of the virus. Drug resistance remains a serious problem. In all likelihood, we'll continually need to cycle in new drugs until we create one capable of clearing the virus once and for all. In other words, until we find a cure.

Treatment faces many obstacles in the places where it's needed most—developing countries, and particularly sub-Saharan Africa. Problems include the heavy costs and getting drugs to everyone who needs them. The lack of facilities to do laboratory tests on things like CD4 levels. The fact that nations don't have enough physicians trained to treat HIV and AIDS or health care professionals to make sure patients correctly take the drugs. The huge and growing number of infected human beings. The difficulty in overcoming cultural obstacles like shame and prejudice and women's low status.

It's possible that the solution to HIV, if one exists, rests with a vaccine.

After the discovery of human immunodeficiency virus in 1984, it seemed only a matter of time before science applied the same technologies to HIV that provided safe vaccines for once-feared killers like smallpox and measles. Margaret Heckler, head of the U.S. Department of Health and Human Services, stated the world would have a vaccine in two years.

The scientists standing near her reacted with stunned expressions. Rightly, as it turned out. More than twenty years later, the world is still waiting, with no end to the search in sight.

Timeline of Research

1986   First reports that azidothymidine (AZT) slowed the progression of AIDS in some patients.

1987   Burroughs Wellcome cuts AZT's cost by 20 percent in response to criticism over prices.

1988   Food and Drug Administration announces new regulations to speed up the approval process for AIDS drugs.

1992   Government institutes the parallel track policy, allowing AIDS patients access to a new medication as early as possible during the drug's development.

1994   AZT approved for pregnant women.

1995   Approval of the first protease inhibitor.

1995-
1996   Breakthroughs in combination therapies.

2001   Thirty-nine drug makers drop lawsuit against South Africa over plans to manufacture and import generic copies of HIV/AIDS medicines.

2006   Development of the first single-pill, once-a-day HIV drug.

2007   Brazil issues compulsory license for the AIDS drug Efavirenz.

six

Today's Pandemic

I f HIV/AIDS exploded on the world in 1981, we're still living within the shockwave as the disease spreads further. From its murky origins in central Africa, HIV has become a pandemic—a worldwide outbreak of infectious disease. Cases have been reported in Greenland, on South Pacific islands, in isolated North Korea. But in recent years the virus has expanded most dramatically on the world's most populous continent—Asia.

Widespread AIDS struck Thailand earlier than it did other Asian nations. The social problems linked to HIV elsewhere allowed the disease a foothold and contributed to its spread.

Thailand entered the 1980s with one of the world's largest sex industries. Fifteen percent of Thai women were sex workers at some point in their lives. In some parts of the country, such work was encouraged as a means to bring in money for a woman's family. Thai culture historically allowed men to have multiple sex partners without shame or stigma. In addition, the industry attracted a significant number of foreign tourists.

Intravenous drug use was also a major problem. Myanmar, Thailand's western neighbor, produced and exported a large amount of the world's heroin. Thailand served as both a market for the drug and as part of the pipeline that shipped it everywhere.

Despite government attempts to discourage contact with foreigners, HIV entered the country in the 1980s. Initial programs were aimed at people engaged in the recognized risk groups—sex workers, IV drug users, and men involved in sexual relationships with other men. At the same time, the government assured Thais outside these groups that AIDS was not a threat to them.

The number of cases climbed dramatically. The rate among IV drug users skyrocketed to 40 percent in under two years. Sex workers in Chang Mai, the major northern city and a center for recruiting sex workers, had HIV-positive rates that were equal and possibly higher.

The 143,000 new cases reported in 1991 looked like the beginning of a disaster. International health experts foresaw a day just ten years later when the country would have 4 million citizens with HIV.

New political leadership looked at the problem and acted. Anand Panyarachun became prime minister in 1991 and immediately made AIDS a public health priority. AIDS activist and politician Mechai Viravaidya, a member of Panyarachun's cabinet, led an information blitz that blanketed Thai pop culture with posters, newspaper advertisements, radio spots, and television messages. Schools were ordered to teach AIDS education. The government gave away free condoms. Later, mothers received AZT to prevent them from passing HIV to their newborns.

It worked. The millions of HIV cases never materialized. According to the World Health Organization estimates, 580,000 Thais had HIV in 2005. New cases were down by 10 percent from the year before.

Experts and officials throughout the world have hailed the Thai effort. Recent complacency, however, threatened to undo the progress. "People think because they can't see HIV anymore that we have it kicked, and they are taking risks again," said Mechai Viravaidya in 2004.

After an economic crisis in the late 1990s, Thailand's government cut condom programs and no longer spent money on its mass media campaign. Promiscuity and unsafe sex rose again. The availability of combination therapy, and the subsequent misconception that it provided an easy treatment for the disease, figured in the change in attitudes, as well.

And many women are being infected by their spouses. In 2005, Thailand's public health ministry estimated that husbands passing the virus to their wives caused one out of three new HIV infections.

While Thailand had success, its neighbors often fared worse.

Myanmar had a huge heroin problem and so little money for health care that hospitals failed to screen blood supplies for HIV.

Vietnam's HIV rate doubled between 2000 and 2005, driven by the same risk behaviors behind its spread elsewhere. In Cambodia, rates seemed to decline in the late 1990s, but statistics are hard to come by.

Laos stood out as an exception. Despite being surrounded by nations with epidemics, Laos has thus far avoided one

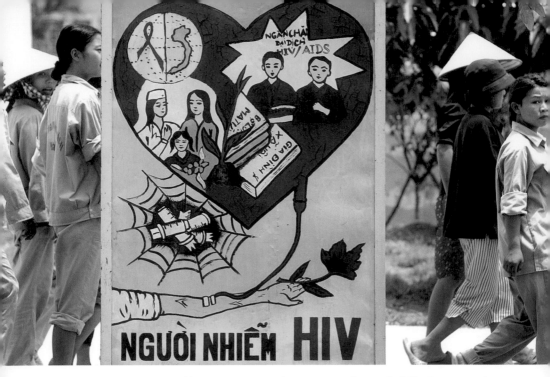

Vietnamese women walking past an AIDS poster at a drug rehabilitaion center in 2004. Vietnam's HIV rate doubled between 2000 and 2005, a surge caused by the same behaviors behind its spread elsewhere in the world. *(Courtesy of AP Images/Richard Vogel)*

of its own. The total number of cases remains unclear due to a lack of research. By 2005, however, the government counted around 1,800 cases, much lower than in neighboring countries.

Laos's isolation and cultural mores may have protected it initially. But a rise in risky behavior and general lack of awareness about the disease present challenges. So does the inadequate medical system. As of 2005, only one hospital in the entire country had access to HIV drugs.

HIV in Thailand's giant neighbor to the north was another matter.

Intravenous drug use powered China's epidemic. Heroin smuggled over the border from Myanmar had turned the southern province of Yunnan into China's center for IV drug use as early as 1989. A little more than ten years later, a United Nations report suggested between 50 and 80 percent of Yunnan's IV drug users were HIV-positive.

Drug-fueled epidemics also appeared elsewhere. Xinjiang, a heavily Islamic province in the far west, borders Afghanistan, another major drug producer. The province had 10 percent of all AIDS cases in China at the end of 2006.

China's epidemic paralleled the worldwide AIDS crisis in other familiar ways, too.

For instance, the country's economic boom encouraged tens of millions of workers to leave rural areas for jobs in the cities. As in Africa, huge numbers of male workers live in dormitories or sleep in shifts in tiny apartments shared with others like them. As in Africa, some of these men pay sex workers, with now-familiar consequences related to HIV.

There are differences, however. For example, women migrate for work almost as often as men. In some provinces, a third of migrant workers take their partners with them. And studies suggest more negative attitudes toward casual sex reduce the number of people exposed to the virus.

While China's HIV problem shaped up in familiar ways, one of its largest epidemics had a more unusual origin.

About 100 million people live in Henan, making it the country's most-populated province. The economic boom that swept so much of China has yet to raise Henan from its status as one of the country's poorest and more rural regions.

In the late 1980s, Henan officials came up with a way to relieve the region's poverty. They encouraged local people to sell plasma, a blood product, for money. Farmer-entre-preneurs acted as brokers between local people and plasma buyers.

Selling plasma was popular. A villager could make a week's wage for about 1.6 pints. The entrepreneurs soon came up with a way of extracting plasma and re-injecting the remaining blood cells back into the donor. That allowed the donor to give plasma multiple times per day without becoming sick.

Selling blood products became a vital part of Henan's economy. "We would sell extra if there was a marriage cer-emony coming up or if we wanted to build a house," said one farmer from Xiongqiao. "The most I ever did was four dona-tions in a single day."

For the most impoverished, the money went toward food and other essentials.

Henan provided a significant amount of China's plasma by the mid-1990s. The money to be made encouraged the industry to barrel ahead without regard for safety. The people in charge of collection, nicknamed "bloodheads," pooled blood products to process the plasma more efficiently and cheaply. As a result, the red and white blood cells re-injected into a donor was not just his or her blood, but that of everyone in the pool.

Blood cells carry HIV. If there was one HIV-positive per-son in the pool, everyone selling plasma that day could get the virus.

AIDS devastated Henan. Cone-shaped mounds of soil marked thousands of graves in fields once used to raise crops. Donors passed the virus to spouses, adding to the death toll. UNICEF estimated that the province had 2,000 AIDS orphans.

The government first responded by covering up. Outside visitors, both Chinese and foreigners, were banned from hard-hit areas. Newspapers fired Chinese journalists digging into the story.

AIDS activists were harassed, even beaten. Gao Yaojie, a physician who helped link the disease to the plasma industry, spent more than ten years being threatened, watched, and listened to by policemen, and occasionally placed under house arrest. As late as 2007, the government refused to let her go to Washington, D.C., to accept an award. (The authorities later relented.)

The Chinese government long refused to admit AIDS had entered the country. Even as the situation in Henan became an emergency and the disease spread in other parts of the country, officials denounced AIDS as a Western problem caused by decadent habits.

It took until 2002 for the government to provide statistics that outside sources considered realistic. That summer, the United Nations released a long report that condemned China's response

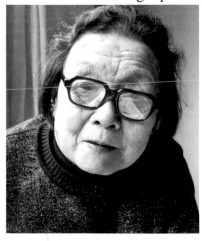

Gao Yaojie, the physician who helped link AIDS to the plasma industry in China's Henan province *(Courtesy of AP Images)*

to HIV/AIDS and compared its leaders to the officers of the famously doomed ship, the *Titanic*. The Chinese dismissed the accusations.

Since then, though, the country has taken steps to address the disease. In 2003, China's leader, Wen Jiabao, signaled a change in the government's attitude by shaking hands with Sun Fuli, an HIV-infected patient at an AIDS treatment center.

Funding for information campaigns and drug treatment programs increased. The government soon announced the "Four Frees and One Care Policy," a treatment and prevention program rolled out in selected parts of the country through 2005.

Under the program, the government gave HIV drugs to low-income patients and to pregnant women and their newborns, provided free testing and counseling, allowed AIDS orphans to attend school for free, and approved financial help for households dealing with the disease. In 2006, about one out of every four people was getting the necessary treatment.

But the effectiveness of this and other anti-HIV policies has been mixed. Ordinary citizens distrust the central government due to its long history of cover-ups, corruption, and outright deception. Local officials have at times blocked or undercut AIDS efforts, sometimes because of worries about image, sometimes because admitting an HIV problem risks losing investment money, sometimes because religious or cultural factors that make them unwilling to consider certain kinds of prevention.

Prejudice also remains a serious problem throughout society. "I asked my mother and relatives in another village if my younger daughter could live with them," an HIV-positive woman in Henan said, "but they refused to take her because they're scared of AIDS—even though my daughter isn't infected. People in other villages are afraid of us. They don't want to talk to us. They won't sit next to us. They don't want to buy vegetables from us."

Doctors, even hospitals, turned away AIDS patients. A survey of health professionals in Yunnan revealed that 30 percent would refuse to treat someone with the disease.

The WHO and China's health ministry estimate that about 650,000 Chinese have HIV. Both admit the number may be as high as more than 1 million. Critics suggest even that number may be too low.

China's difficulty in addressing AIDS makes some experts worry its situation may eventually resemble that of sub-Saharan Africa. Given China's population of 1.3 billion human beings, even an epidemic that struck 1 percent of the country's people would equal a staggering 13 million infections.

The fear of HIV loose in a large population also comes into play in India.

India recorded its first AIDS case in 1986. The next year the government started its first program to take charge of the country's response. It evolved into the National AIDS Control Organisation, in 1992.

A worker receives an HIV test for free at a construction site in China's Henan province. Although China has taken steps to address the AIDS epidemic, the effectiveness of its anti-HIV policies remains unproven. *(Courtesy of AP Images)*

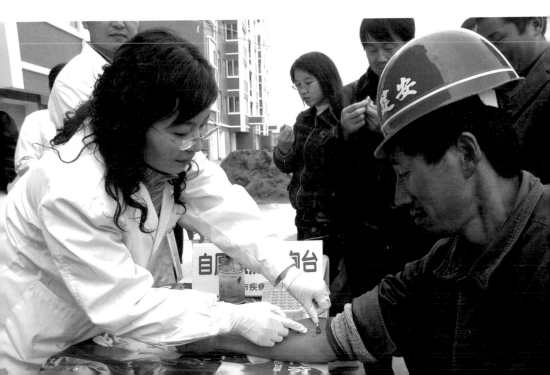

Despite improved blood screening and other measures, however, HIV skipped out of India's risk groups and into the general population. The 200,000 cases estimated in 1990 grew to 3.9 million cases at the end of the decade. From 2000 to 2003, the number rose to 5.1 million, with huge gains among young and middle-aged adults. That was greater than the number of HIV-positive people in Thailand, Myanmar, Laos, Cambodia, and Vietnam combined.

India's crisis is complex. The country's size and enormous population allow it to sustain what are really a number of separate epidemics, each with its own character.

In some cities, for instance, HIV got its start among urban sex workers. But IV drug users represent the most numerous victims in areas bordering Myanmar. Workers migrating for jobs, gay men, the poor—all are represented in varying numbers and in different ways depending on where they live.

There's mobility. As happens in Africa, HIV rates soar along the large highways connecting the major cities of New Delhi, Calcutta, Chennai, and Mumbai—what Indians called the Golden Quadrilateral. Hundreds of thousands of trucks crisscross the country carrying goods. By 2005, one in ten truckers was estimated to be HIV-positive. The drivers passed the virus to their spouses or other partners, as did workers migrating back and forth from villages to India's cities looking for jobs.

There's prejudice. An HIV-positive Indian faces beatings, denial of care, loss of employment, and banishment from his or her family. Not surprisingly, fear keeps most HIV-positive Indians from seeking medical care. The WHO estimated that only 7 percent of those who need drug therapy got it. Even

India's status as a source of generic HIV medicines hasn't done much to boost the treatment rate.

There's a huge population of poor people. Fear of persecution isn't the only thing preventing proper medical care. Tens of millions of Indians suffer from extreme poverty. Many don't live near a treatment center and can't afford to make regular train trips if it is a long distance away.

The Indian government has added to the confusion by periodically backing away from the problem. For example, the Health Ministry counted 520,000 new HIV infections in 2003. The next year, the Indians reported a mere 28,000. Regions wracked with HIV and AIDS one year before now claimed to have no cases at all. No international organization believed the numbers.

Getting an accurate estimate remains a problem today. In 2007, the United Nations estimated India had 5.7 million people living with HIV. If true, that placed the country first in total HIV cases, ahead of South Africa. The Indian government, however, stated it was 5.2 million cases, or just behind South Africa.

Then a new study made the situation even murkier. While the report remained unpublished and therefore unofficial, it revised the number of HIV-infected Indians to between 2 and 3 million, far below other estimates.

Asia isn't the only new AIDS frontier. In recent years, the pandemic has struck again in Europe, as Russia and Ukraine struggle to get a handle on their outbreaks.

The fall of the Soviet Union in the early 1990s plunged the Russian Federation into continuous economic problems. The resulting poverty and hopelessness drove many Russians to substance abuse. Escalating IV drug use, combined with

RIGHT: An Indian sex worker demonstrates how to use a condom during an AIDS prevention training session in Mumbai, India. *(Courtesy of Indranil Mukherjee/APF/ Getty Images)*

BELOW : Truck drivers listen to an AIDS prevention volunteer near a highway in Gauhati, India. *(Courtesy of AP Images/ Anupam Nath)*

the collapse of the country's public health system, paved the way for risk behaviors associated with HIV while at the same time crippling the institutions set up to deal with the threat of infectious disease.

Statistics in Russia are untrustworthy, making it hard to measure HIV's spread. A 2007 report counted 402,000 cases, with 17,000 deaths. But the numbers leaned heavily on people who had been tested already. The World Health Organization estimates the number at around 940,000. Russia's own AIDS officials say it may be closer to 1.3 million while the WHO and UN put the possible top figure at 1.6 million.

HIV in Russia is a disease of the young. Statistics suggest that four of every five people living with the virus are between fifteen and thirty years old.

It also follows economic development. In a few Russian cities, a stunning 10 percent of adult men carry HIV. That's consistent with United Nations data that shows the virus has hit hardest in wealthy and more developed regions, especially urban areas.

Intravenous drug users remain most at risk, but the new cases in that group have declined. Now that HIV and AIDS have reached saturation, the disease has crossed over into the heterosexual population.

The number of infected women is on the rise. So are the number of AIDS orphans. Many are newborns abandoned by substance-abusing parents. Because test kits for HIV are rare and expensive, the nurses caring for the children cannot be sure the infants are HIV-positive at all.

Regions on the country's outskirts, like Chechnya in southern Russia, have reported their own outbreaks. The 1990s civil war destroyed Chechnya's public health infrastructure and forced thousands of soldiers and refugees to fan out into neighboring countries. War and mobile populations, as so often happens, encouraged HIV's spread.

Until recently, international agencies considered Ukraine's epidemic in its early stages, as those infected tended to belong to the well-known risk groups. But since 2004, tests have shown a spike in people infected through heterosexual contact. In fact, Ukraine had one of the highest infection rates for pregnant women in Europe by 2006.

The government moved to give anti-HIV medication to mothers and newborns. As a result, fewer children are born with the virus than before. But agencies had trouble finding all HIV-positive women in time to give them treatment.

As HIV has expanded its reach, fallout from the disease—stigmatization and economic distress, to name two things—have become social and economic issues in their own right. What's sometimes overlooked is that the spread of the virus has influenced a surge in other infectious diseases that have been with us far longer than HIV.

In the U.S., for instance, hepatitis C—a disease with no cure or vaccine—often piggybacks on HIV infection.

An HIV-positive mother in Kiev, Ukraine, cuddles her two-month-old baby girl in this 2005 photo. The woman said she contracted the disease from her late husband, who was a drug user. The baby has not tested positive for the disease. *(Courtesy of Brent Stirton/Getty Images for GBC)*

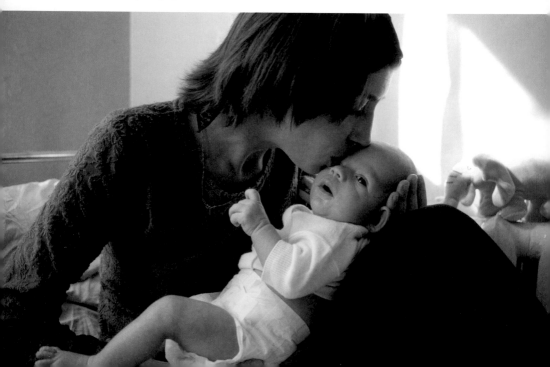

The true global threat of the moment, however, comes from tuberculosis.

Tuberculosis is a contagious respiratory disease. Historically, it's aggravated by hunger, substance abuse, exposure to the elements, and several other environmental conditions common to the poor. It had a heyday in the 1800s, when the smoky air and backbreaking labor of the Industrial Revolution gave it huge populations to infect.

Though treatable in the twentieth century, TB lingered in a large part of the world. HIV and AIDS have now opened the door to new and more intense epidemics.

Tuberculosis is the number one opportunistic infection among sub-Saharan Africa's HIV-positive adults. Many people there live with inactive TB present in their body. HIV's attack on the immune system boosts the tuberculosis bacterium's ability to reproduce. Active tuberculosis follows. One disease multiplies the effects of the other and the immune system collapses as it's tag-teamed by the two deadly diseases.

HIV has helped encourage tuberculosis to mutate into strains unaffected by most drugs used to treat it, leaving patients even more vulnerable.

It's now a cliché that HIV is the most-studied virus in human history. The hard truth is that the research and scholarship will probably continue for a long time. The horrible situation in sub-Saharan Africa, the ominous epidemic in India, and the likely spread into Eastern Europe from Russia show the disease continues its relentless march.

In fact, we're having trouble stopping it despite all our study and research, despite the recognition of risk groups and ten years of miraculous drugs. And even if a vaccine appeared tomorrow, getting it to those in need would take billions of dollars—a financial hurdle that already keeps us from getting malaria drugs and polio vaccine to large parts of the developing world.

There is hope, however. Infection rates in teens and children have gone down in hard-hit countries like Côte d'Ivoire, Malawi, and Zimbabwe. China's government has intervened in some regions with successful information and safe sex campaigns. The World Health Organization reported that in 2006 more than 2 million people in low- and middle-income nations had access to treatment, an all-time high.

There is also a greater financial commitment. The administration of President George W. Bush promised billions of dollars to fight the disease in Africa. The U.S. government now devotes considerable amounts of money for research on HIV vaccines, a notable change from the past.

A number of foundations, including organizations led by former president Bill Clinton and Microsoft founder Bill Gates, continue to raise money and awareness. Movements to address issues related to AIDS, like the relationship between African poverty and foreign debt, have gained attention.

But the problem is immense.

AIDS was the first major infectious disease to emerge in the modern era of advanced science, mass media, and international institutions. The epidemics and the pandemic that followed have taught us a lot—about ourselves and the world and our vulnerability to new and undiscovered viruses.

Where HIV leads, and whether its lessons help us with the next disease to appear, remains to be seen.

Sources

INTRODUCTION

p. 11, "Throughout history . . ." Committee on World
Food Security, "The impact of HIV/AIDS on food security,"
Food and Agricultural Organization of the United
Nations, May 28, 2001, http://www.fao.org/DOCREP/
MEETING/003/Y0310E.HTM.

CHAPTER ONE: The Virus

p. 13, "There's no reason . . ." Mary Carmichael, "How it
began: HIV before the age of AIDS," Frontline,
May 30, 2006, http://www.pbs.org/wgbh/pages/frontline/
aids/virus/origins.html.

CHAPTER TWO: The Emerging Epidemic

p. 28, "The thing that annoys me . . ." John-Manuel Andriote,
Victory Deferred: How AIDS Changed Gay Life in America
(Chicago: University of Chicago Press, 1999), 16.

p. 29, "total body rot . . ." Jonathan Engel, *The Epidemic:
A Global History of AIDS* (New York: Smithsonian
Books, 2006), 7.

p. 30, "I think there was certainly . . ." Ronald Bayer and
Gerald M. Oppenheimer, *AIDS Doctors: Voices from
the Epidemic* (New York: Oxford University Press,
2000), 21.

p. 31, "It's genocide . . ." Elinor Burkett, *The Gravest Show
on Earth* (Boston: Houghton Mifflin, 1995), 288.

p. 33, "I am angry and frustrated . . ." Larry Kramer, "1112
and counting," from *Reports from the Holocaust* (New
York: St. Martin's Press, 1994), p. 44.

p. 42, "political meddlers," Robert Pear, "AIDS at 20: Advocates for patients barged in, and the federal government changed," *New York Times*, June 5, 2001.

CHAPTER THREE: Fear, Loathing, and Change

p. 46, "perverse homosexuals . . ." Andriote, *Victory Deferred*, 68.

p. 47, "If you brought up . . ." Bayer and Oppenheimer, *AIDS Doctors: Voices from the Epidemic*, 108.

p. 53-54, "Do as little as possible . . ." Randy Shilts, *And the Band Played On* (New York: St. Martin's Press, 1987), 527.

p. 55, "They didn't back down . . ." *Nation*, "ACT UP at 20," editorial, April 9, 2007, http://www.thenation.com/doc/20070409/act_up.

p. 59,61, "[E]ven as far back . . ." Linda Villarosa, "A conversation with Phill Wilson: Speaking out to make AIDS an issue of color," *New York Times*, December 19, 2000, http://query.nytimes.com/gst/fullpage.html?sec=health&res=9905E7DD1239F93AA25751C1A9669C8B63.

p. 61-62, "Whether it is a teen . . ." Leslie Fulbright, "Disease denial devastating for African Americans," *San Francisco Chronicle*, June 5, 2006, http://sfgate.com/cgi-bin/article.cgi?f=/c/a/2006/06/05/AIDSBLACK.TMP.

CHAPTER FOUR: "Slim"

p. 66, "I couldn't believe . . ." Laurie Garrett, *The Coming Plague: Newly Emerging Diseases in a World Out of Balance* (New York: Penguin Books, 1994), 338.

p. 74, "I didn't break down . . ." Jonathan Mann and Daniel Tarantola, eds., *AIDS in the World II* (New York: Oxford University Press, 1996), 349.

p. 80, "behaved angrily . . ." IRIN, "Kenya: Protecting widows from dangerous customs," United Nations Office for the Coordination of Humanitarian Affairs, June 19, 2007, http://www.plusnews.org/report.aspx?ReportID=72821.

p. 81, "The policies for orphans . . ." Lawrence K. Altman, "African grandmothers rally for AIDS orphans," *New York Times*, August 13, 2006.

CHAPTER FIVE: The Treatment Revolution

p. 88, "Today's approval . . ." Food and Drug Administration, news release, March 20, 1987, http://www.fda.gov/bbs/topics/NEWS/NEW00217.html.

p. 88, "I never quit . . ." Susan Hunter, *AIDS in America* (New York: Palgrave Macmillan, 2006), 185.

p. 91, "For the first time . . ." Frontline, "Interview David Ho," May 30, 2006, http://www.pbs.org/wgbh/pages/frontline/aids/interviews/ho.html.

p. 102, "a landmark for those suffering . . ." Marc Kaufman, "FDA clears once-a-day AIDS drug," *Washington Post*, July 13, 2006, http://www.washingtonpost.com/wp-dyn/content/article/2006/07/12/AR2006071201172.html.

p. 103, "We are still . . ." Luc Montagnier and Stephen Sartarelli, trans., *Virus* (New York: W. W. Norton, 2000), 147.

CHAPTER SIX: Today's Pandemic

p. 107, "People think because . . ." Christine Gorman, "Sex, AIDS, and Thailand," *Time*, July 12, 2004, http://www.time.com/time/magazine/article/0,9171,501040719-662826,00.html.

p. 110, "We would sell extra . . ." Jonathan Watts, "Hidden

from the world, a village dies of AIDS while China refuses to face a growing crisis," *Guardian (London)*, October 25, 2003, http://www.guardian.co.uk/china/story/0,7369,1070800,00.html.

p. 112, "I asked my mother . . ." UNICEF, "China's children affected by HIV/AIDS," http://www.unicef.org/china/reallives_588.html.

Bibliography

BOOKS

Allen, Peter Lewis. *The Wages of Sin: Sex and Disease, Past and Present*. Chicago: University of Chicago Press, 2000.

Andriote, John-Manuel. *Victory Deferred: How AIDS Changed Gay Life in America*. Chicago: University of Chicago Press, 1999.

Ashe, Arthur, and Arnold Rampersad. *Days of Grace*: *A Memoir*. New York: Ballantine Books, 1994.

Burkett, Elinor. *The Gravest Show on Earth*. Boston: Houghton Mifflin, 1995.

Clarke, Loren K., and Malcolm Potts, eds. *The AIDS Reader*. Boston: Branden Publishing, 1988.

d'Adesky, Anne-Christine. *Moving Mountains: The Race to Treat Global AIDS*. New York: Verso, 2004.

Epstein, Helen. *The Invisible Cure*. New York: Farrar, Straus, Giroux, 2007.

Garrett, Laurie. *Betrayal of Trust: The Collapse of Global Public Health*. New York: Hyperion, 2000.

———. *The Coming Plague: Newly Emerging Diseases in a World Out of Balance*. New York: Penguin Books, 1994.

Grmek, Mirko D., Russell C. Maulitz, and Jacalyn Duffin, trans. *History of AIDS: Emergence and Origin of a Modern Pandemic*. Princeton, NJ: Princeton University Press, 1993.

Hunter, Susan. *AIDS in America*. New York: Palgrave Macmillan, 2006.

———. *AIDS in Asia: A Continent in Peril*. New York: Palgrave Macmillan, 2005.

————. *Black Death: AIDS in Africa*. New York: Palgrave Macmillan, 2003.

Karlen, Arno. *Man and Microbes*. New York: G. P. Putnam's Sons, 1995.

Kinsella, James. *Covering the Plague: AIDS and the American Media*. Piscataway, NJ: Rutgers University Press, 1989.

Kramer, Larry. *Reports from the Holocaust*. New York: St. Martin's, 1994.

Levenson, Jacob. *The Secret Epidemic: The Story of AIDS and Black America*. New York: Pantheon, 2004.

Mann, Jonathan, and Daniel Tarantola, eds. *AIDS in the World II*. New York: Oxford University Press, 1996.

McNeill, William H. *Plagues and Peoples*. Garden City, NY: Anchor Press/Doubleday, 1976.

Montagnier, Luc, and Stephen Sartarelli, trans. *Virus*. New York: W. W. Norton, 2000.

Nolen, Stephanie. *28 Stories About AIDS in Africa*. New York: Walker and Co., 2007.

Porter, Roy. *The Greatest Benefit to Mankind*. New York: W. W. Norton & Company, 1997.

Rosen, George. *A History of Public Health*. Baltimore, MD: Johns Hopkins University Press, 1993.

Shilts, Randy. *And the Band Played On*. New York: St. Martin's Press, 1987.

Smith, Raymond A., ed., *Encyclopedia of AIDS*. New York: Penguin, 2001.

Starr, Douglas. *Blood: An Epic History of Medicine and Commerce*. New York: Knopf, 1998.

PERIODICALS

Altman, Lawrence K. "African grandmothers rally for AIDS orphans." *New York Times*, August 13, 2006.

———. "Chimp virus is linked to HIV." *New York Times*, May 26, 2006.

———. "Troubling side effects are linked to effective AIDS therapy." *New York Times*, July 7, 1998.

Burr, Chandler. "The AIDS exception: Privacy vs. public health." *Atlantic Monthly* 279, no. 6 (June 1997): 57–67.

Cohen, Jon. "A new treatment campaign, but with limited weapons." *Science* 304, no. 5676 (June 4, 2004): 1433–1434.

———. "An unsafe practice turned blood donors into victims." Ibid., 1438–1439.

———. "Asia and Africa: On different trajectories?" *Science* 304, no. 5679 (June 15, 2004): 1932–1938.

———. "Changing course to break the HIV-heroin connection." *Science* 304, no. 5676 (June 4, 2004): 1434–1435.

———. "Poised for takeoff?" Ibid., 1430–1432.

Diamond, Bruce. "Debate escalates on source of sub-Saharan Africa's AIDS epidemic." *Nature Medicine* 10, no. 5 (May 2004): 441.

Gill, Bates, and Susan Okie. "China and HIV—A window of opportunity." *New England Journal of Medicine* 356, no. 18 (May 3, 2007): 1801–1805.

Gottlieb, M. S., and H. M. Schanker, et. al. "*Pneumocystis* pneumonia—Los Angeles," *Morbidity and Mortality Weekly Report* 30, no. 21 (June 5, 1981): 1–3.

Marantz Henig, Robin. "A new disease's deadly odyssey." *New York Times Magazine*, February 6, 1983.

Kolata, Gina. "The genesis of an epidemic: Humans, chimps, and a virus." *New York Times*, September 4, 2001.

———. "Hit hard by AIDS virus, hemophiliacs angrily speak out." *New York Times*, December 25, 1991.

———. "On research frontier, basic questions." *New York Times*, June 5, 2001.

————. "When HIV made its jump to people." *New York Times*, January 29, 2002.

Koup, Richard A. "A new latent HIV reservoir." *Nature Medicine* 7, no. 4 (April 2001): 404–405.

Montagnier, Luc. "A history of HIV discovery." *Science* 298, no. 5599 (November 29, 2002): 1727–1728.

Navarro, Mireya. "Children with a secret (spelled AIDS)." *New York Times*, March 28, 1991.

Pear, Robert. "AIDS at 20: Advocates for patients barged in, and the federal government changed." *New York Times*, June 5, 2001.

Power, Samantha. "The AIDS rebel." *New Yorker*, May 19, 2003.

Rosenberg, Tina. "Look at Brazil." *New York Times Magazine*, January 28, 2001.

Schneider, E., and M. K. Glynn, et. al. "Epidemiology of HIV/AIDS—United States, 1981–2005." *Morbidity and Mortality Weekly Report* 55, no. 21, 589–592.

Stotto, Michael A. "The precautionary principle and emerging biological risks: Lessons from swine flu and HIV in blood products." *Public Health Reports* 117 (November/December 2002): 546–552.

Villarosa, Linda. "One disease, live six different ways." *New York Times*, June 5, 2001.

Waldholz, Michael. "Some AIDS cases defy new drug 'cocktails.'" *Wall Street Journal*, October 10, 1996.

Waldman, Amy. "On India's roads, cargo and a deadly passenger." *New York Times*, December 6, 2005.

Zeeman, Beth. "HIV-AIDS in Tanzania—realities on the ground." *New England Journal of Medicine* 355, no. 22, 2276–2277.

ONLINE

Adams, Brad, and Joanne Csete, et. al, eds. "Locked Doors: The human rights of people living with HIV/AIDS in China." Human Rights Watch publication, August 2003. http://www.hrw.org/reports/2003/china0803/.

Amaral, Ricardo. "Brazil bypasses patent on Merck AIDS drug." Reuters, May 4, 2007. http://www.alertnet.org/thenews/newsdesk/N04351721.htm.

Batty, David. "The battle for cheap AIDS drugs." *Guardian (London)*, May 9, 2007. http://www.guardian.co.uk/aids/story/0,,2075950,00.html.

Becker, Jasper. "China becomes proactive." *San Francisco Chronicle*, February 9, 2003. http://sfgate.com/cgi-bin/arti

Bell, Thomas. "Nepal facing AIDS epidemic." *San Francisco Chronicle*, February 24, 2003. http://sfgate.com/cgi-bin/article.cgi?file=/chronicle/archive/2003/02/24/MN146530.DTL.

Boustany, Nora. "Group honors doctor who exposed China AIDS scandal." *Washington Post*, March 15, 2007. http://www.washingtonpost.com/wp-dyn/content/article/2007/03/14/AR2007031402699.html.

Brodie, Mollyann, and Elizabeth Hamel, et. al. "AIDS at 21: Media coverage of the HIV epidemic 1981–2002." Kaiser Family Foundation publication no. 7023. http://www.kff.org/kaiserpolls/upload/AIDS-at-21-Media-Coverage-of-the-HIV-Epidemic-1981-2002-Supplement-to-the-March-April-2004-issue-of-CJR.pdf.

Bronski, Michael. "Rewriting the script of Reagan: why the president ignored AIDS." *Forward,* November 14, 2003. http://www.forward.com/articles/rewriting-the-script-on-reagan-why-the-president/.

Centers for Disease Control. "HIV/AIDS among African Americans." CDC fact sheet, June, 2007. http://www.cdc.gov/hiv/topics/aa/resources/factsheets/pdf/aa.pdf.

Brown, David. "AIDS study focuses on 'elite controllers.'" *Washington Post*, August 17, 2006. http://www.washingtonpost.com/wpdyn/content/article/2006/08/16/AR2006081601484.html.

Clarke, Jeremy. "African AIDS victims fret over India patent case." Reuters, March 5, 2007. http://www.alertnet.org/thenews/newsdesk/L23415113.htm.

Committee on World Food Security. "The impact of HIV/AIDS on food security." Food and Agricultural Organization of the United Nations, May 28–June 1, 2001. http://www.fao.org/DOCREP/MEETING/003/Y0310E.HTM.

Daley, Suzanne. "Runaways of 42^d street: AIDS begins its scourge." *New York Times*, May 30, 1988. http://query.nytimes.com/gst/fullpage.html?sec=health&res=940DEFD7103DF933A05756C0A96E948260.

Dodge, Willian IV. "Living with HIV in the U.S." *Frontline: The Age of AIDS*, undated. http://www.pbs.org/wgbh/pages/frontline/aids/past/liveus.html.

Drevna, Darryl, Leslie Isenegger, and Amanda Wolfe. "*Kaiser Daily HIV/AIDS Report* looks at twenty years of legislation and policy." *Kaiser Daily HIV/AIDS Report*, June 7, 2001. http://www.kaisernetwork.org/daily_reports/rep_index.cfm?DR_ID=5036.

Dries-Daffner, Ingrid, Melissa Keefe, and Meredith Weiner. "*Kaiser Daily HIV/AIDS Report* looks at how early confusion over AIDS created stigmas." *Kaiser Daily HIV/AIDS Report*, July 5, 2001. http://www.kaisernetwork.org/daily_reports/rep_index.cfm?DR_ID=4981.

Eberstadt, Nicholas. "The future of AIDS." *Foreign Affairs*, November/December 2002. http://www.foreignaffairs.org/20021101faessay9990/nicholas-eberstadt/the-future-of-aids.html.

Economist. "Blood debts." January 18, 2007. http://www.
economist.com/world/asia/displaystory.cfm?story_id=
8554778.

Epstein, Helen. "Africa's lethal web net of AIDS." *Los Angeles
Times*, April 15, 2007. http://www.latimes.com/
news/opinion/la-op-epstein15apr15,0,5804078.
story?coll=la-opinion-rightrail.

———. "God and the fight against AIDS." *New York
Review of Books*, April 28. 2005. http://www.nybooks.
com/articles/17963.

———. "Why is AIDS worse in Africa?" *Discover*, February
5, 2004. http://discovermagazine.com/2004/feb/why-
aids-worse-in-africa.

Faulconbridge, Guy. "Russia warns of AIDS epidemic, 1.3
million with HIV." Reuters, May 15, 2007. http://www.
reuters.com/article/healthNews/idUSL1546187520070515.

Frankel, Rafael D. "Burma's leaders slowly moving to
combat HIV." *San Francisco Chronicle*, April 3, 2003.
http://sfgate.com/cgi-bin/article.cgi?file=/chronicle/
archive/2003/04/03/MN212143.DTL&type=health.

French, Howard W. "China's Muslims awake to nexus of
needles and AIDS." *New York Times*, November 12, 2006.
http://www.nytimes.com/2006/11/12/world/asia/12
aids.html?ex=1185422400&en=23adf587cb4a0275&ei=
5070.

Fulbright, Leslie. "Disease denial devastating for African
Americans." *San Francisco Chronicle*, June 5, 2006.
http://sfgate.com/cgi-bin/article.cgi?f=/c/a/2006/06/
05/AIDSBLACK.TMP.

Gallagher, John. "The hope whisperer." *Advocate*, July
21, 1998. http://findarticles.com/p/articles/mi_m1589/is_
n764/ai_20944421.

Gifford, Rob. "One man against AIDS in China." National Public Radio, All Things Considered (transcript), July 26, 2005. http://www.npr.org/templates/story/ story.php? storyId=4772130.

Golden, Frederic. "The first chimpanzee." *Time*, February 8, 1999. http://www.time.com/time/magazine/article/ 0,9171,19538,00.html.

Gonzalez, David. "Looking past fear of AIDS to see a child." *New York Times*, December 3, 1996. http://query.nytimes. com/gst/fullpage.html?sec=health&res=9C05E3D8103C F930A35751C1A960958260.

Gorman, Christine. "Sex, AIDS, and Thailand." *Time*, July 12, 2004. http://www.time.com/time/magazine/article/ 0,9171,501040719-662826,00.html.

Gorst, Isabel. "Russia: The trouble with a patriarchal society." *Financial Times*, December 1, 2006. http://www.ft. com/cms/s/a7ebe31c-78bc-11db-802c-0000779e2340, dwp_uuid=727810ac-7ef7-11db-b193-0000779e2340.html.

Henkel, John. "Attacking AIDS with 'cocktail' therapy." *FDA Consumer*, July-August 1999. http://www.fda.gov/ fdac/features/1999/499_aids.html.

Hilts, Philip J. "Drug said to help AIDS cases with virus but no symptoms." *New York Times*, August 18, 1989. http://query.nytimes.com/gst/fullpage.html?sec=health& res=950DE3DA153FF93BA2575BC0A96F948260.

IRIN staff. "Kenya: Protecting widows from dangerous customs." *PlusNews*, June 19, 2007. http://www.plusnews. org/report.aspx?ReportID=72821.

———. "Laos: Keeping the lid on HIV." *Reuters AlertNet*, January 30, 2007. http://www.alertnet.org/thenews/ newsdesk/IRIN/e4e0323ebd9da3c86f691179fe5d594a.htm.

———. "New thinking needed on 'AIDS orphans.'" United Nations Office for the Coordination of Humanitarian

Affairs, October 30, 2003. http://www.irinnews.org/
report.aspx?reportid=46986.

————. "Swaziland: New HIV/AIDS support programme
unveiled for truckers." United Nations Office for
the Coordination of Humanitarian Affairs, June 1, 2007.
http://www.irinnews.org/Report.aspx?ReportId=72503

Jack, Andrew, and Richard Lapper, "Brazil overrides
Merck patent on AIDS drug." *Financial Times*, May 4,
2007. http://www.ft.com/cms/s/c7d3f1f4-fa78-11db-8bd0-
000b5df10621.html.

Johnson, Jo. "India: A threat to economic ambition."
Financial Times, December 1, 2006. http://www.ft.com/
cms/s/85edbda6-7bb1-11db-b1c6-0000779e2340,dwp_
uuid=727810ac-7ef7-11db-b193-0000779e2340.html.

Joint United Nations Programme on HIV/AIDS (UNAIDS)
and World Health Organization. "AIDS epidemic update:
December 2006." UNAIDS document no. 06.29E,
December, 2006. http://www.who.int/hiv/mediacentre/
2006_EpiUpdate_en.pdf.

Kaiser Family Foundation. "Black Americans and HIV/
AIDS." Kaiser Family Foundation publication no. 6089-04,
July, 2007. http://www.kff.org/hivaids/upload/6089-04.pdf.

————. "The multisectoral impact of the HIV/AIDS
epidemic, a primer." Kaiser Family Foundation publication
no. 7661, July, 2007. http://www.kff.org/hivaids/upload/
7661.pdf.

Kaiser Daily HIV/AIDS Report. "Number of HIV/AIDS
cases in Russia increasing, health official says." *Kaiser
Daily HIV/AIDS Report*, May 17, 2007. http://www.
kaisernetwork.org/Daily_reports/rep_index.
cfm?DR_ID=44962.

Kates, Jennifer, Annette Martin, and Alicia Carbaugh.
"HIV/AIDS in India." Kaiser Family Foundation

publication no. 7312-003, September, 2006. http://www.kff.
org/hivaids/upload/7312-03.pdf

Kates, Jennifer, and Alyssa Wilson Leggoe. "The HIV/
AIDS epidemic in Malawi." Kaiser Family Foundation
publication no. 7359, October, 2005. http://www.kff.
org/hivaids/upload/7359.pdf.

————. "The HIV/AIDS epidemic in Swaziland."
Kaiser Family Foundation publication no. 7366,
October, 2005. http://www.kff.org/hivaids/upload/7359.
pdf.

————. "The HIV/AIDS epidemic in the United Republic
of Tanzania," Kaiser Family Foundation publication no.
7367, October, 2005. http://www.kff.org/hivaids/upload/
7367.pdf.

Kaufman, Marc. "FDA clears once-a-day AIDS drug."
Washington Post, July 13, 2006. http://www.washington
post.com/wpdyn/content/article/2006/07/12/AR
2006071201172.html.

Koop, C. Everett. "Understanding AIDS." U.S. Department
of Health and Human Services. HHS Publication No.
(CDC) HHS-88-8404. May 4, 1988. http://profiles.
nlm.nih.gov/QQ/B/D/R/L/.

LaFraniere, Sharon. "New AIDS cases in Africa outpace
treatment gains." *New York Times*, June 6, 2007. http:
//www.nytimes.com/2007/06/06/health/06aids.
html?ex=1184990400&en=144c642dce5cadf1&ei=5070.

Lerner, Sharon. "Black women and HIV." *Village Voice*,
July 19, 2000. http://www.villagevoice.com/
news/0029,lerner,16559,5.html.

McGreal, Chris. "AIDS: South Africa's new apartheid."
Guardian (London), November 30, 2000. http://www.
guardian.co.uk/aids/story/0,7369,405587,00.html.

McLaughlin, Abraham. "Africa fights AIDS with girl power." *Christian Science Monitor*, December 17, 2004. http://www.csmonitor.com/2004/1217/p06s01-woaf.html.

————. "For AIDS orphans, lessons on life—and car repair." *Christian Science Monitor*, February 23, 2006. http://www.csmonitor.com/2006/0223/p01s04woaf. html?s=hns.

McNeil, Donald G. Jr. "India, said to play down AIDS, has many fewer with virus than thought, study finds." *New York Times*, June 8, 2007. http://www.nytimes. com/2007/ 06/08/world/asia/08aids.html?ex=1338955200&en= c20701f60f5af445&ei=5088&partner=rssnyt&emc= rss.

————. "Made in India, a favored 'cocktail' for AIDS." *New York Times*, May 4, 2004. http://query.nytimes.com/ gst/fullpage.html?res=9F06E4D7133DF937A35756C0A962 9C8B63&sec=health.

Mydans, Seth. "Dying in Vietnam, they are ignored but trying to laugh." *Boston Globe*, June 5, 2006. http://www. boston.com/yourlife/health/diseases/articles/2006/06/ 05/dying_in_vietnam_they_are_ignored_but_trying_ to_laugh/.

Nation. "ACT UP at 20." April 9, 2007. http://www.thenation. com/doc/20070409/act_up.

National Institutes of Health. "In their own words: NIH researchers recall the early years of AIDS." Undated. http://history.nih.gov/NIHInOwnWords.

New York Times. "Finding virus in wild chimp advances hunt for source of AIDS." January 18, 2002. http://query. nytimes.com/gst/fullpage.html?sec=health&res= 9A05EEDA1E38F93BA25752C0A9649C8B63&n=Top% 2fNews%2fHealth%2fDiseases%2c%20Conditions%2c %20and%20Health%20Topics%2fAIDS.

Park, Alice. "China's secret plague. *Time*, July 19, 2004. http:/ /www.time.com/time/magazine/article/0,9171,557111, 00.html.

Pepper, Daniel. "Follywood." *POZ*, July/August 2007. http:// www.poz.com/articles/2023_12131.shtml.

Perry, Alex. "When silence kills." *Time*, May 30, 2005. http:// www.time.com/time/magazine/article/0,9171,1066961-2,00.html.

Peterson, Scott. "On front line of AIDS in Russia." *Christian Science Monitor*, August 17, 2004. http://www.csmonitor. com/2004/0817/p07s01-woeu.html.

———. "Reluctantly, Russia confronts AIDS." *Christian Science Monitor*, August 16, 2004. http://www.csmonitor. com/2004/0816/p06s01-woeu.html.

Pocha, Jehangir S. "Heroin, ignorance boost spread of AIDS in Chinese province." *Boston Globe*, June 5, 2006. http:// www.boston.com/yourlife/health/diseases/ articles/2006/06/05/heroin_ignorance_boost_spread_ of_aids_in_chinese_province/.

———. Transcript of interview with Li Dan. *Boston Globe*, March 27, 2006. http://www.boston.com/news/world/ asia/articles/2006/03/28/transcript_of_interview_with_ li_dan/.

Rainsford, Sarah. "Russia's AIDS timebomb." *British Broadcasting Corporation*, December 3, 2003. http://news. bbc.co.uk/2/hi/europe/3284141.stm.

Reel, Monte. "Where prostitutes also fight AIDS." *Washington Post*, March 2, 2006. http://www.washingtonpost.com/ wp-dyn/content/article/2006/03/01/AR2006030102316_ pf.html.

Rosenthal, Elizabeth. "AIDS scourge in rural China leaves villages of orphans." *New York Times,* August 25, 2002. http://query.nytimes.com/gst/fullpage.html?sec=health& res=9E04EED9133CF936A1575BC0A9649C8B63.

Russell, Sabin. "New crusade to lower AIDS drug costs. *San Francisco Chronicle*, May 24, 1999. http://sfgate. com/cgibin/article.cgi?file=/chronicle/archive/1999/05/ 24/MN104738.DTL.

Shapiro, Nina. "The new faces of AIDS." *Seattle Weekly*, October 24, 2002. http://www.alternet.org/story/14372/.

Silvers, Jonathan. "Orphaned by AIDS." *Online Newshour* (transcript), May 9, 2002. http://www.npr.org/templates/ story/story.php?storyId=4772130.

Smith, Stephen. "AIDS drug's high costs spurs doctors' boycott." *Boston Globe*, March 19, 2004. http://www. boston.com/news/nation/articles/2004/03/19/aids_ drugs_high_cost_spurs_doctors_boycott/.

Stolberg, Sheryl Gay. "Bush requests $30 billion to fight AIDS." *New York Times*, May 31, 2007. http://www. nytimes.com/2007/05/31/washington/31prexy. html?ex=1185422400&en=a2a8d31933c4b4a6&ei=5070.

Swarns, Rachel L. "Drug makers drop South Africa suit over AIDS medicine." Associated Press, April 20, 2001. http://query.nytimes.com/gst/fullpage.html?sec=health& res=9F00E6DE1330F933A15757C0A9679C8B63.

Terzieff, Juliette. "Pakistani woman battles AIDS stigma in her country." *San Francisco Chronicle*, November 17, 2002. http://sfgate.com/cgi-bin/article.cgi?file= /c/a/2003/03/22/MN156716.DTL&type=health.

Timberg, Craig. "Spread of AIDS in Africa is outpacing treatment." *Washington Post*, June 20, 2007. http://www. washingtonpost.com/wp-dyn/content/article/2007/06/ 19/AR2007061901971.html.

UNICEF. "China's children affected by HIV/AIDS." UNICEF document, undated. http://www.unicef.org/china/reallives_ 588.html.

————. "Kindergartens help care for abandoned babies as AIDS epidemic grows." UNICEF document, February 9, 2005. http://www.unicef.org/infobycountry/russia_25079.html.

————. "Orphans and other children affected by HIV/AIDS." UNICEF document, September, 2003. http://www.unicef.org/publications/files/Orphans_and_Other_Children_Affected_by_HIV_AIDS.pdf.

Vanage, Gavin du. "AIDS orphans strain South Africa." *San Francisco Chronicle*, July 11, 2002. http://sfgate.com/cgi-bin/article.cgi?f=/c/a/2002/07/11/MN38988.DTL.

Villarosa, Linda. "A conversation with Phill Wilson: Speaking out to make AIDS an issue of color." *New York Times,* December 19, 2000. http://query.nytimes.com/gst/fullpage.html?sec=health&res=9905E7DD1239F93AA25751C1A9669C8B63.

Watts, Jonathan. "Hidden from the world, a village dies of AIDS while China refuses to face a growing crisis." *Guardian (London)*, October 25, 2003. http://www.guardian.co.uk/china/story/0,7369,1070800,00.html.

Wines, Michael. "AIDS blamed for legions of orphans in Africa." *New York Times*, November 27, 2003. http://query.nytimes.com/gst/fullpage.html?sec=health&res=9501E0DB173AF934A15752C1A9659C8B63.

World Health Organization. "Global AIDS epidemic continues to grow." World Health Organization news release, November 21, 2006. http://www.who.int/hiv/mediacentre/news62/en/index.html.

————. "Significant growth in access to HIV treatment in 2006." World Health Organization news release, April 17, 2007. http://www.who.int/mediacentre/news/releases/2007/pr16/en/index.html.

World Health Organization, UNAIDS, and UNICEF. "Toward universal access: Scaling up priority HIV/AIDS interventions in the health sector, progress report, April 2007." World Health Organization, April 2007. http://www.who.int/hiv/mediacentre/universal_access_progress_report_en.pdf.

Wright, Kai. "Black, gay, at-risk." *Village Voice*, June 21, 2000. http://www.villagevoice.com/news/0025,wright2,15804,5.html

———. "Emergency call." *Village Voice*, June 14, 2000. http://www.villagevoice.com/news/0024,wright,15637,5.html.

Yardley, Jim. "China covers up detention of AIDS doctor." *New York Times*, February 16, 2007. http://www.nytimes.com/2007/02/16/world/asia/16china.html?ex=1329282000&en=32541f3224d8060c&ei=5088&partner=rssnyt&emc=rss.

Web Sites

http://www.cdc.gov/hiv/default.htm
The Centers for Disease Control is the jumping off point for all information related to HIV/AIDS in the United States, and on this site, visitors will find a wealth of information on HIV prevention and treatment.

http://www.amfar.org/cgi-bin/iowa/index.html
Founded in 1985, the Foundation for AIDS Research (amfAR) is working to find solutions to end the global AIDS epidemic through innovative research. A short video on this site details the organization's work.

http://www.unaids.org/en/
Links to the most current news worldwide, speeches, major events, and publications are available on this Web site, which is maintained by the Joint United Nations Program on HIV/AIDS (UNAIDS).

http://www.kff.org/hivaids/index.cfm
An interactive Web-based timeline of key HIV-related events and noteworthy activities from 1981 through today is one of the best features of this Kaiser Family Foundation site.

Glossary

asymptomatic
Showing no outward signs (symptoms) of disease.

CD4 positive (CD4+) T-cells
The CD4 positive (CD4+) T-cell helps direct the immune system's response to an invading virus, bacterium, or other agent. HIV attacks these cells. The level of these cells in the body is one of the factors used to determine if a patient has progressed to AIDS.

clade
A family of genetically similar viruses.

combination therapy
Combination therapy is the use of several drugs to simultaneously attack different aspects of HIV in order to stop or reverse its progress.

drug resistance
Drug resistance in HIV occurs when the virus changes its genetic structure via mutation into forms that are no longer affected, or as affected as before, by medication.

epidemic
An epidemic is a higher-than-usual number of cases of a disease in a population.

hemophilia
Hemophilia is an inherited disorder, most often affecting males, that prevents the blood from clotting properly.

pandemic
A series of epidemics taking place over a large area of the world.

syphilis
A sexually-transmitted disease caused by the corkscrew-shaped bacterium *Treponema pallidum*. Syphilis was first recorded in Europe in 1493 and may have originated in the New World.

urbanization
Urbanization is the process of an individual, group, or society joining in an urban (usually as opposed to a rural) way of life. Often used to mean the mass migration of rural people to cities.

Index